Tl

Fibromyalgia
Dental
Handbook

FLORA PARSA STAY, DDS, holds a doctor of dental surgery degree from the University of California, San Francisco. She is the developer of Grace Fibro-Smile, a line of dental care products for those with fibromyalgia, available on her web site, www.drstay.com. She is the author of *The Complete Book of Dental Remedies* and contributing author to *Women and Health, Herbal Health, Health and Aging,* and *Natural Prescriptions for Women.* She has written for or been interviewed in many publications, including *Prevention, Men's Health, Women's World,* the *Ventura County Star,* and the *New York Times.* She runs a private practice in Ventura, California, where she lives with her husband.

The
Fibromyalgia
Dental
Handbook

A Practical Guide to
Maintaining Peak Dental Health

FLORA PARSA STAY, DDS

FOREWORD BY R. PAUL ST. AMAND, MD

MARLOWE & COMPANY
NEW YORK

THE FIBROMYALGIA DENTAL HANDBOOK:
A Practical Guide to Maintaining Peak Dental Health
Copyright © 2005 by Flora Parsa Stay
Foreword copyright © 2005 by R. Paul St. Amand

Published by
Marlowe & Company
An Imprint of Avalon Publishing Group Incorporated
245 West 17th Street • 11th Floor
New York, NY 10011-5300

AVALON
publishing group incorporated

LIBRARY OF CONGRESS CATALOGING-IN-PUBLICATION DATA
Parsa Stay, Flora.
The fibromyalgia dental handbook : a practical guide to maintaining peak dental health /
by Flora Parsa Stay ; foreword by R. Paul St. Amand.
p. cm.
Includes bibliographical references and index.
ISBN 1-56924-401-4 (pbk.)
1. Mouth—Care and hygiene—Popular works. 2. Fibromyalgia—Popular works.
3. Mouth—Diseases—Popular works. I. Title.
RK61.P263 2005
617.5'22—dc22
2005000879

9 8 7 6 5 4 3 2 1

Designed by Pauline Neuwirth, Neuwirth & Associates
Printed in the United States of America

I dedicate this book to the millions of people living with fibromyalgia who live courageously through physical, mental, and emotional adversity above the disbelief of others about their illness. Never give up. You are my heroes.

Contents

Foreword

by R. Paul St. Amand, MD

Enlightenment is education. Medicine is no different in that regard than is electronic technology. Advancing the scope of science usually comes in nibbles and bite-sized revelations. Rarely does a huge, new morsel get downed all at one time and even then it is on the shoulders of what went before. Knowledge evolves from basic research as an accumulation of seemingly unrelated facts. Sooner or later an individual or team coordinates them and new realizations surface.

So it is that fibromyalgia is not a new disease. It has always plagued the human race, unfortunately too often ascribed to a psychological base. When hypochondriasis was first challenged and a physical illness suggested, rejection was swift. Could something so extensive in the population really exist, nameless, through the millennia? But stubbornness is a quality of all great scientists and several of them persisted until a syndrome was clearly defined. Only twenty years later, it's now conceded that fibromyalgia affects between five and fifteen percent of the female population. Even the low-end estimate translates into several hundred million people worldwide who suffer from this (in historical terms) newly named entity.

In this book, Dr. Flora Parsa Stay helps us discover more important facts in our ongoing quest towards fully understanding fibromyalgia. In keeping with her dental versatility, she dares to tell us that there is a connection between the oral cavity, the brain, the musculoskeletal system, and the irritable bowel syndrome common to fibromyalgia. In a strange coincidence, my initial encounter with this unknown disease began in the mouth when a patient of mine suggested his gout medication was allowing dental calculus (tartar) to crumble off his teeth. He wasn't wrong. Forty-five years later, this expert on oral disease reminds us that the head bone is indeed connected to the toe bone.

When I first met Flora, she was already known for her pioneering spirit in rejecting conventional wisdom. She was truly one of the first to realize that what is used in the mouth is absorbed into the bloodstream and can have an effect on the whole body. Her concern about additives in toothpastes led her to design her own for her patients. Her previous book of dental remedies underscored her commitment to safe, simple solutions when big manufacturers refused to see the need or respond. When I found it necessary to tell my patients to avoid certain chemicals—salicylates—a Google search led me to Flora and the products featured on her Web site. Her response was instant, helpful, and wise. Together we have learned from each other and expanded each other's knowledge. I've recently read in medical journals facts that Flora provided to me long ago. Apparently what she told me then is conventional wisdom now!

Luckily for humanity, there are those who commit to freely use their expertise and help others. Dr. Parsa Stay and her husband, Andy, have contributed greatly to ease the way for individuals with fibromyalgia. Her Web site and newsletter have reached many without charge. Flora and Andy have created a multitude of high quality, safe, salicylate-free products, much to the relief of those using my guaifenesin protocol. Her concern about each and every ingredient they contain is inspiring. They have also given significant sums to promote research in the field. She now adds this book as further testimony to her unwaning dedication to finding solutions for this major problem. I commend you, Flora. Thanks for contributing to an unfinished story.

R. PAUL ST. AMAND, MD, has been on the teaching staff at the Los Angeles Harbor/UCLA Hospital, Department of Endocrinology for over forty-five years and is the coauthor of *What Your Doctor May Not Tell You About Fibromyalgia*. He lives in Los Angeles.

Introduction

What's this all about?

I hope this book will provide a powerful tool to help you understand how your oral health affects your fibromyalgia and many of its symptoms. I want to empower you to learn how poor dental health can have a daily effect on fibromyalgia. I want to help you learn to manage your oral health well so you can avoid these problems and feel better and healthier. As you learn more about the importance of your oral health to you as a person who deals with the fibromyalgia every day, you will be better prepared to work with your dentist to eliminate any oral issues that may aggravate your condition. As you'll soon see, oral problems are important because they can relate directly to digestive problems, muscle pain, and many other symptoms common to people with fibromyalgia. As a result of what you'll learn by reading this book, your mouth will be healthier, and you will be confident that you have one less factor contributing to fibromyalgia symptoms.

A Bit of Background

When I graduated from the University of California at San Francisco School of Dentistry in 1975, no one knew anything about fibromyalgia. Over the years, as more people cried out to their physicians with similar symptoms, a specific diagnosis began to emerge and a name had to be found to identify this group of physical complaints. By the late 1980s, **fibromyalgia syndrome (FMS)** became recognized as a condition with a particular set of recurring symptoms.

About ten years ago, I began to notice that many of my dental patients who told me that they had fibromyalgia tended to have certain oral issues in common, but I couldn't find anything in the medical or dental professional literature that gave me much insight into aspects of fibromyalgia that were related to oral health. Clearly something was missing and I began to think about finding that missing link.

As my fibromyalgia patient base continued to increase, I continued to think about the recurrent dental problems that I was seeing in this group. I began to read everything I could get my hands on concerning fibromyalgia. My conclusion: there is an important connection between oral health and fibromyalgia symptoms and, conversely, poor oral health can greatly worsen the already very difficult problems associated with the disease.

Fibromyalgia and Dental Health

The word *fibro* means fibrous tissue (tendons and ligaments), and *myalgia* refers to muscle pain. A national support group called the Fibromyalgia Network defines fibromyalgia as a widespread musculoskeletal pain and fatigue disorder for which the cause is still unknown. Painful muscles are felt mostly in the shoulders, buttocks, neck, lower back, and jaw. Although its causes are still uncertain, fibromyalgia appears in an estimated two to four percent of the general population—perhaps ten million people nationally. Fibromyalgia affects more women than men, but occurs in every age group.

We now know that everything in the body is connected. Even how we think about our health can impact our well-being. But did you ever consider that the health of your mouth could affect how your whole body feels and could affect the management of fibromyalgia?

As someone suffering with fibromyalgia, you probably have experienced health concerns in nearly every part of your body, including your mouth. Most patients with fibromyalgia say that they ache all over, with muscles that feel like they have been pulled or overworked. Their muscles sometimes twitch; sometimes there is an unpleasant burning sensation.

Part of the difficulty in understanding fibromyalgia is that it displays so many symptoms that frequently differ from person to person. Although not everyone has all of these problems associated with fibromyalgia, several of them frequently occur at once and you have probably experienced many of them.

- Fatigue is present in varying degrees, from mild to severe. Many people report difficulty concentrating and experience short-term memory loss ("brain fog").
- Musculoskeletal pain is another common symptom, with sensations described deep aching, burning, and shooting pain. The pain is pinpointed in tender "trigger points" which are anatomically defined. The pain may feel worse in the morning and result in stiffness, especially in muscle groups that are used most often.
- Insomnia is a common complaint among people with fibromyalgia, most of whom have no problems falling asleep, but don't reach deep sleep (Level Four) long enough to get needed rest and rejuvenation.
- Depression is often present, but may be due to dealing with fibromyalgia and not necessarily a cause of it.

◆ Chronic headaches, such as migraines and tension headaches are noted in about fifty percent of patients.
◆ **Temporomandibular joint disorder (TMJ)** is accompanied by severe pain in the jaw, face, and neck. This may cause difficulty chewing, yawning, and even talking. Approximately

Here is a quick reference list of some of the most common problems associated with fibromyalgia:

Pain in the muscles and soft tissues
Morning stiffness
Chronic fatigue
Painful menstruation
Sleep disruption
Chronic headaches
Irritable bowel syndrome
Dizziness
Depression and anxiety
Exercise intolerance
Cognitive or memory impairment
Lessened ability to concentrate
Problems performing multiple tasks at one time
Numbness and tingling sensations
Muscle twitching and muscle weakness
Irritable bladder
Bloating, gas, belching, pain, and distension
The feeling of swollen extremities
Skin sensitivities
Dry eyes and mouth
Frequent changes in eye prescription
Impaired coordination
Chronic runny nose

seventy percent of fibromyalgia patients report jaw pain of varying degrees. TMJ has many other symptoms including dizziness, headaches, pain in neck, shoulder, and back pain, headaches, and ringing in the ears.

◆ **Irritable bowel syndrome** is found in about forty to seventy percent of people with fibromyalgia, and causes constipation, diarrhea, gas, abdominal pain, and nausea.

◆ Dry eyes and mouth are often experienced among those with fibromyalgia.

◆ Numbness and tingling sensations in the hands and feet are sometimes noted by people with fibromyalgia.

Several of these symptoms are related directly to your oral health, including irritable bowel syndrome, TMJ, and several others.

Irritable Bowel Syndrome and the Mouth

Irritable bowel syndrome (IBS) is a common chronic disorder of the large intestine that causes a host of nasty problems, including abdominal pain, bloating, gas, cramping, diarrhea, and constipation. These symptoms are often brought on by eating a large amount of food, alcohol, caffeine, chocolate, carbonated drinks, and fatty foods. There is no cure for irritable bowel syndrome, but to manage it and prevent breakouts of symptoms, treatment involves diet changes, medication, and stress management—and often some actions to improve your dental health.

While we don't understand all the causes irritable bowel syndrome, we do know that digestion begins in the mouth and that an unhealthy mouth can lead to unhealthy digestion. If your fibromyalgia includes digestive problems, your mouth is the logical place to start. If you have missing or painful teeth or other oral problems, it is virtually impossible to chew food properly and adequately. Improper chewing, in turn, affects your ability to absorb food and determines the extent to which undigested food is stored and eliminated by the large intestine. If you can't handle the initial phases of digestion properly, your colon will not function as it should. The result can be the symptoms common to irritable bowel syndrome.

It is interesting that the same foods that bring about symptoms related to irritable bowel syndrome will also cause dental problems. Drinking too much alcohol dries the mouth and may cause gum disease, sores, and oral cancer. Carbonated drinks are full of sugar and acid, and cause cavities and eroded **enamel**. The same is true with frequent consumption of simple carbohydrates, which will cause cavities as well as gas and bloating in irritable bowel syndrome.

In a nutshell, then, if you have poor oral health, possibly made worse by some dietary mistakes, you may be undermining your ability to digest your food and triggering irritable bowel syndrome.

Fibromyalgia, Facial Pain, and TMJ

If your fibromyalgia is fairly typical, you have to deal with aching or burning muscles and joints just about every day. These painful trigger points may show up in the same muscle groups or vary in location throughout your body.

You may get considerable relief from painful muscles and joints with weekly or even daily visits to the chiropractor or physical therapist. However, TMJ may not lend itself to these treatments—not if the problem stems from dental health. This syndrome targets the muscles and ligaments surrounding the jaw. This syndrome causes tremendous face and head pain in one quarter of the population who have fibromyalgia. Studies have shown that up to ninety percent of people with fibromyalgia have jaw and facial tenderness that could produce symptoms of TMJ .

If your upper and lower jaws are not aligned properly, chiropractic adjustments will not hold and, very quickly after treatment by a chiropractor, the muscle and joints begin to hurt again. The balance of the musculoskeletal system cannot be maintained for long if an underlying imbalance in the jaw is not addressed. What's worse, these biomechanical issues can cause pain to radiate from your jaw to the head, neck, shoulder, back, and even the calves.

Other Important Connections

Medical science is finally taking notice that this organ we call the **oral cavity** is more than just teeth that need to be drilled and filled. We now know that gum disease will increase the risk of stroke, heart disease, and low birth weight of premature babies. A diseased mouth can also adversely affect diabetes and increase the risk of lung disease. In fact, there is a wide and sometimes surprising range of connections between oral health and the body's overall condition.

For example, obesity has also been connected to high risk of heart disease, and now even to gum disease. It all makes sense when you consider that except for obesity due to a medical condition, a person who is obese gained weight from eating foods that were not very nutritious, and from eating excessively. Studies indicate that certain vitamins and minerals are extremely important to the health of the gums and teeth. Vitamin C deficiency will lead to bleeding gums. Calcium deficiency can result in weak teeth. A diet high in sugar and junk foods will lead to cavities and gum disease. There is a high incidence of cavities and gum disease in obese individuals.

Recent medical reports state that gum inflammation (**gingivitis**) may be an important contributoto hardening of the arteries. When there is tissue damage in the body, such as inflammation, organs send out chemical signals indicating something is abnormal. **C-reactive protein (CRP)** is one such marker for inflammation in the body. Elevated c-reactive protein has been linked to heart attacks, strokes, and peripheral arterial disease.

There are many more important connections, as you'll learn in the pages ahead. Most specifically—and this is the whole point of my writing and your reading this book—there are many links between oral health and FMS. The more you learn about the subject, the better you will grasp the interconnectedness of the many aspects of oral health (or problems) and FMS symptoms.

What You Will Find in This Book

This book is organized into nineteen chapters that cover all pertinent topics about FMS as it relates to oral health. As best I am aware, it is a completely unique book on this subject. In the pages that follow, you will find discussions on everything from nutritional considerations to sleep disorders to fluoridation to coping with feelings of fear and anxiety that many people experience when they visit the dentist's office. I have tried to be concrete and practical about every topic, and wherever possible I have offered suggestions for techniques, activities, and products that will be of use to you. I have also added information about various theories and treatments associated with holistic dentistry, even though, as you will read, I am very skeptical about the scientific basis or effectiveness of much of this sort of therapy.

While I have tried to be comprehensive in selecting subject material, I have worked hard to keep the special interests and needs of my readers in mind; every chapter relates not only to an oral health topic, but also to its direct relationship to FMS. Above all else, my intention has been not merely to inform you, but to supply you with the tools and knowledge to improve your health and your life.

While I encourage you to read the entire book in the order written, I have developed each chapter so that it forms a complete, independent unit, with all the facts and explanation needed to form a freestanding discussion. This way you will be able to read chapters with subjects of special importance to you before reading the rest of the book.

A note about technical terms: I wrote this book for people who have fibromyalgia or who have a family member or friend with that disease. I don't expect you to have a clinical or scientific background and I have kept the material in the book as simple, non-technical, and reader-friendly as I could. Even so, I have had to use some technical terms to explain a variety of topics related to fibromyalgia. As you'll see throughout the book, whenever I use a technical term for the first time, the word is set in **boldface type**. This indicates that a definition of the word appears in the glossary at the back of the book. More than likely, if you encounter an unfamiliar technical term at any point in the text, the glossary will provide its definition.

Some other resources: Please note that, along with the glossary, the back sections of the book include a "Dental Problem Guide," that I've designed as a quick reference to help readers prepare for and deal with dental emergencies; a listing of suggested reading categorized by specific topics, and a list of additional sources of information and support.

1

GUM AND BONE

Building Strong Foundations

> The wise man built his house on rock. The rain fell,
> the floods came, and the winds blew and buffeted the house.
> But it did not collapse; it had been set solidly on rock . . .
> But the fool built his house on sand. The rain fell, the floods
> came, and the winds blew and buffeted the house.
> And it collapsed and was completely ruined.
> —*Matthew 7:24*

According to the Food and Drug Administration, more than seventy-five percent of Americans over the age of thirty-five have some form of gum disease. This may be because this is a silent disease, giving no obvious symptoms or pain until it's too late. Because it doesn't give any advanced notice of its presence, unless you're aware of the early signs that accompany **periodontal (gum) disease,** you may eventually lose your teeth. Bad as that is, research studies have reported that there is more at risk than losing teeth to gum disease.

Untreated, gum disease can lead to:

◆ Increased risk of heart disease
◆ Increased risk of stroke
◆ Exacerbation of diabetes
◆ Respiratory diseases
◆ **Osteoporosis**
◆ Pre-term or low birth weight babies

Gum disease is common in people with fibromyalgia for several reasons. Far too often, it may simply be that people with fibromyalgia have so many health issues to deal with that early warning signs of gum disease are ignored. Your fibromyalgia also makes you much more subject to chronic **dry mouth**, which can aggravate **plaque** build-up, the greatest source of gum disease. So, sad to say, you are at greater risk of developing gum disease than people who do not have fibromyalgia. You need to be vigilant to stay ahead of this serious problem.

Bleeding When You Brush Is Not Okay

Before you learn more about what causes gum disease and how to avoid it, let's discuss how to determine if you have it. There are specific signs that go along with gum disease. Most people know little about these warning signs or when to seek treatment. Following are some questions to ask yourself to determine if you have periodontal (gum) disease:

- Do your gums bleed when you brush or floss?
- Do you have bad breath?
- Do your teeth appear to have spaces between them that were not there before?
- Do you have swollen gums or notice any pus around them?
- Do areas of your gums appear red and feel tender to the touch?
- Does your bite seem changed so that your teeth don't fit or come together evenly?
- Do you get an itchy feeling on the gums?

Put very simply, gum disease is an infection of the tissues and bone that support the teeth. There are millions of bacteria present in the mouth at all times. While many oral bacteria are harmless, some can attack gum and teeth and cause disease. The harmful bacteria thrive in a clear film that accumulates on the teeth and gums, called **plaque**. If plaque is not removed thoroughly on a daily basis but instead is left unchecked, it will destroy bone and connective tissue, resulting in teeth become loose and ultimately might need to be pulled.

Gum disease is related to age less than people think and is the most frequent cause of losing teeth. Why is someone with fibromyalgia prone to developing gum disease? As I've stated already, plaque build up is the most frequent cause of gum disease, and plaque builds up more aggressively due to dry mouth—a common, daily problem among many people with fibromyalgia. Other causes of gum disease include:

♦ Poor diet—Foods high in sugar deprive the body of vital nutrients that help ward off gum disease. Vitamin C and **antioxidants** are very important for healthy tissues in the mouth, as is a balanced diet rich in fruits and vegetables. If your diet is too high in sugar or too low in the right nutrients, you increase your risk of gum problems. It is also believed foods high in simple carbohydrates such as sugar may worsen fibromyalgia symptoms.

The May 2003 issue of the *Journal of Periodontology* reported a study from Case Western Reserve University of 13,700 individuals that found a relationship between obesity and gum disease. Obese individuals had a seventy-five percent higher incidence of **periodontal disease** than people of normal weight. The diet of the obese people contained fewer vegetables and fruits. A diet that is not balanced increases the chance for gum disease.

Calcium is another important nutrient because healthy bone is needed to support and maintain the teeth, and diets low in calcium are more likely to cause gum disease and bone loss. For people with low calcium intake, the risk for gum disease increases to fifty-four percent and for those with moderate calcium intake, it increases by approximately twenty-seven percent. Calcium is also important in proper muscle function, which is crucial if you have TMJ (see Chapter Three) or if muscular pain is a symptom of your fibromyalgia.

◆ Stress—There is no quicker path to ill health, including gum disease, than failing to cope with stress. Stress management is very important in maintaining good health. Stress makes it harder for the body to avoid infection. Because fibromyalgia may be an **autoimmune disorder** (it has yet to be proven), excessive stress makes it harder for the body to repair and heal itself.

◆ Smoking—All tobacco products predispose a person to gum disease, mainly because smoking dries the mouth and deprives the tissues of vital rebuilding nutrients. Your fibromyalgia already causes your mouth to be dry; smoking makes the problem worse—besides posing many other very serious hazards.

◆ Genetics—Approximately thirty percent of the population is likely to develop gum disease due to heredity.

◆ Depression—Alarmingly common in fibromyalgia, depression also increases the risk of gum disease. A University of North Carolina study published in the April 2002 issue of the *Journal of Periodontology* concluded that depression weakens the immune system, thereby affecting the body's ability to heal and maintain the health of gums. Additionally, individuals who are depressed may be less concerned with taking care of themselves and may allow their health to deteriorate. In addition, many medications prescribed for depression result in dry mouth as a side effect.

◆ Poor **oral hygiene**—Within six hours after the teeth are cleaned plaque returns. Within twenty-four to thirty-six hours, this thin film of food and bacteria begins to cause gum inflammation. The amount of bacteria present and the strength of the body's natural defense mechanism or resistance to disease will determine how rapidly periodontal disease advances.

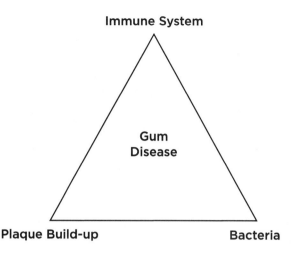

Figure 1 The area where all three factors overlap is when the most destruction of the supporting structures of the teeth occurs.

◆ Hormonal changes—During puberty, pregnancy, and menopause, people experience many hormonal fluctuations. If proper oral hygiene is not maintained during these periods, gum disease can result.

◆ Poorly maintained fillings—Old, fractured, rough or leaky fillings offer a trap for bacteria and can spread disease in the mouth.

◆ **Clenching** or grinding the teeth—This may cause **gum recession**, which can lead to gum disease.

◆ Medication—Some drugs cause dry mouth, thereby leading to gum disease, while others such as infertility treatment drugs, result in a higher incidence of gingival inflammation and progression of gum disease. (This relationship presents something of a "Catch 22," because some studies indicate that chronic inflammation and infection affect reproduction success and infertility treatment.)

◆ Diabetes—People with diabetes are more likely to have gum disease since they are generally prone to infections. In fact, gum disease is the sixth most widespread complication of diabetes. Advanced gum disease can increase blood sugar levels, which can heighten the risk of complications for the diabetic. Studies published in the November 2003 issue of the *Journal of Periodontology* established that individuals with well controlled Type Two diabetes are less prone to gum disease, while those with poorly controlled diabetes are more likely to develop advanced gum disease. Conversely, some studies indicate that chronic gum inflammation (gum disease) increases the risk of developing diabetes.

◆ Contagion—Some types of gum disease are contagious and can be passed through infected **saliva** from parents to children and between adults.

Gum Disease and Heart Disease:
Signs of Heart Disease Most Ignored

There are two theories about the relationship between gum disease and heart disease. One theory holds that bacteria thrive in the gums and cause inflammation. These bacteria enter the blood vessels, attach to fatty plaques in the coronary arteries (those within the heart), and contribute to clot formation. These blood clots constrict the flow of oxygen and nutrients to the heart, thereby causing heart disease and heart attack.

Another theory asserts that gum inflammation and plaque build-up contribute to swelling of the arteries, leading to coronary artery disease. This correlation has been determined through the measurement of C-reactive protein (CRP) levels. Elevated C-reactive protein levels have been found to be important markers for inflammation. C-reactive protein is made by the liver and released in the bloodstream whenever there is inflammation present anywhere in the body. Studies have shown that when C-reactive protein is present in the bloodstream, the risk of heart disease increases. In fact, the presence of C-reactive protein more clearly predicts heart attacks than increased cholesterol levels.

Researchers have now been able to show that the presence of bacterial by-products in advanced gum disease can enter the bloodstream and trigger production of C-reactive protein by the liver. A study of 5,000 adults in the United States was conducted to determine the risk of atherosclerosis. The study confirmed that body mass and periodontal disease both increased levels of C-reactive protein in adults. The conclusion is that people with gum disease have almost twice as great a risk of developing coronary artery disease.

People with heart conditions often must take **antibiotics** before dental treatment, because if bacteria from the mouth enter the bloodstream and travel to the heart, bacterial endocarditis (an infection of the heart) may result, sometimes with fatal results. If you have heart disease, your dentist should consult with your cardiologist to determine if you should take antibiotics prior to dental treatment. This is an important example of why it is so important to let your dentist know all of your health conditions.

What does all this information mean to the person with fibromyalgia? Due to the many health issues that affect someone living with fibromyalgia, the immune system is compromised. With the presence of gum disease, the risk of heart disease is highly increased and must not be ignored. Now that we know gum disease is a form of infection accompanied by inflammation, and the relationship of inflammation to increased presence of C-reactive proteins, it would be truly foolish to ignore the signs and symptoms of periodontal disease.

Stages of Gum Disease

Gum disease is a progressive disease. Up to a certain point, it can be reversed, but once bone loss occurs, it becomes more difficult to cure. With advanced bone loss, it may become irreversible and result in tooth loss. Unfortunately, the progress of the disease gives few obvious warning signs such as pain. However, certain signs do accompany different stages, and are recognizable to those who know what to look for.

First let's consider what healthy gums are like:

- Healthy gums appear pink and firm.
- Brushing or flossing does not cause bleeding.
- Healthy gums follow the contour of the teeth and have a scalloped appearance.

In the gum tissue around each tooth, there is a groove called the *gingival sulcus*. By inserting a periodontal probe in several spots around this groove, the dentist takes and records measurements. The probe has a ruler on one end that allows the dentist to take readings of the health of the bone surrounding the teeth. With normal, healthy gums the readings are no more than three millimeters in depth. When unhealthy, these areas form deep pockets referred to as **periodontal pocket**s.

As gum disease progresses, the following aberrations occur:

Gingivitis. This is the initial stage of gum disease, characterized by:
- There is some bleeding of the gums during brushing or flossing.
- Gums may appear slightly red and tender.
- Bad breath is present.

Mild Periodontitis. The signs that were present in gingivitis become pronounced in this stage:
- Bleeding while brushing or flossing becomes more frequent.
- Gums appear red, swollen, and tender.
- Bad breath and an unpleasant taste in the mouth are present.
- There is some destruction of periodontal attachments

between the teeth and gum, forming periodontal pockets of three to four millimeters in depth. These areas are measured every few months with the periodontal probe and the measurements are recorded for future reference so the healing or advancement of disease can be compared.

Moderate Periodontitis. As gum disease progresses, destruction moves deeper through the bone and tissues:

♦ Gums may recede and pull away from the teeth, so teeth appear longer.

♦ Gum infections in the form of **abscess**es may form.

♦ Bad breath and taste worsen.

♦ Teeth may begin to show spacing and drift; thus the bite doesn't feel normal.

♦ Due to further bone destruction, periodontal pockets measure four to six millimeters.

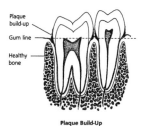

Plaque Build-Up
Direct cause of gingivitis is plaque build-up on teeth at gum line.

Stage 1
Gingivitis, the first stage of gum disease, is characterized by inflamed gums that begin to recede.

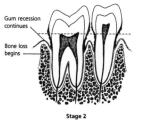

Stage 2
Left untreated, gingivitis develops into periodontitis. During this stage, gums continue to recede and the underlying bone begins to degenerate.

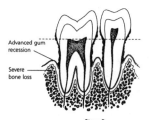

Stage 3
Severe bone loss and gum recession mark advanced periodontitis.

Figure 2 Progression of Periodontal (Gum) Disease.

Advanced Periodontitis. In this stage, the following may occur:

- Teeth may loosen.
- Teeth may have to be extracted, or may fall out on their own.
- Some pain or sensitivity may be felt because receding gums expose teeth **root**s.
- Fever and a general feeling of ill health may occur.
- Periodontal pockets are measured at over six millimeters.

Osteoporosis and Gum Disease

Chronic musculoskeletal pain, depression, and many other features characterize fibromyalgia and appear to have some interrelation, although how these factors are associated is unclear and all are not necessarily present in the same individual. One study on bone mineral density (BMD) revealed a relationship to past or current depression in women and osteoporosis. Researchers then conducted a study to find a connection between BMD and osteoporosis in women with fibromyalgia. Women in the age groups of thirty-three to sixty were evaluated. The study concluded that fibromyalgia was frequently associated with osteoporosis.

One relationship is clear, however: If you have low bone density, or osteoporosis, your chance of having gum disease is increased by more than eighty percent. If the body requires bone tissue, one of the first places from which it leaches tissue is the jaw. With low bone density, the jaw does not provide a strong foundation to support the teeth. Studies published in the *Journal of Periodontology* show hormone replacement therapy can help reverse bone loss. Discussion with your physician will determine if hormone replacement therapy is appropriate for you and what the other options may be. However, if other factors such as good oral hygiene and regular professional cleanings are not kept up, the condition will worsen.

Respiratory Disease and Gum Disease

Harmful bacteria that grow in the mouth, (as in gum disease), and in the throat can be aspirated into the lungs and cause a variety of respiratory diseases such as pneumonia. People with existing respiratory diseases may worsen their conditions with the development of periodontal disease, because their protective immune system is already compromised and weakened. Smoking is a major cause of **chronic obstructive pulmonary disease (COPD)**. If people with chronic obstructive pulmonary disease also have gum disease, they may suffer from bouts of infection due to aspiration of bacteria originating in the mouth. If you have any form of respiratory disease and have dry mouth as a symptom of your fibromyalgia, you will have a tendency to accumulate more plaque. Maintaining a healthy mouth is crucial to your overall health.

Treatment of Gum Disease

As I've indicated, periodontal disease can play a role in heart disease, diabetes, low-birth-weight babies, respiratory disease (bacterial pneumonia), increased risk of stroke, and other health issues. Early detection and treatment of gum disease is vital, especially to the person with fibromyalgia, whose immune system is already compromised by the many health conditions it is trying to resist and overcome.

All stages of gum disease affect the whole body because the disease is essentially a chronic inflammation and/or infection and any such disorder causes detrimental effects throughout the body. With fibromyalgia, you can't help but feel tired and run down if your immune system is not only trying to fight off multiple disorders, but gum disease as well. If your immune system is overburdened in this way, practically any form of treatment for the many health conditions accompanying fibromyalgia will take longer to be effective. Let's consider the ways to treat the several stages of gum disease. Getting these under control will be important for your general well-being and will make efforts to treat your other symptoms quicker and more effective. This will give you the energy and sense of well-being you need to deal with other symptoms of fibromyalgia.

Treatment for Gingivitis

The first step toward treatment is a visit to the dentist. X-rays and pocket depth evaluations will determine if there is loss of bone or destruction of connective tissue attachments. If there is no bone loss, but only presence of inflammation, plaque, and **tartar**, the diagnosis is gingivitis.

Gingivitis is the initial stage of gum disease and is totally reversible. A thorough professional cleaning and daily proper home care will reduce and eliminate all the symptoms. However, visits for professional cleanings and evaluations every four to six months are extremely important; otherwise gingivitis may return and advance to the more destructive stages of gum disease.

Supplements such as calcium, vitamin C, and antioxidants are also useful. Some studies show positive results with **coenzyme Q10** (see page 9) for all stages of gum disease. However, I cannot overstress the importance of regular professional cleanings and daily proper home care, without which all the supplements in the world will be ineffective. In other words, if the bacteria remain and thrive, the disease will advance and destroy tissue, whether you take supplements or not.

Treatment for Mild Periodontitis

With mild periodontitis, there is some destruction of the connective tissue attachments between the teeth and gums. The dentist determines the extent of gum pockets by measuring around each tooth in six specific spots. The readings may vary in some spots from two to four millimeters. The treatment may include any or all of the following:

◆ **Scaling and root planning (SRP)**—The dentist or hygienist cleans under the gums to the depth of the pocket, removing all plaque or **tartar (calculus)**. This may be done with a local or topical **anesthetic**. The whole mouth may be cleaned in one appointment or in two to four appointments, treating one or two "**quadrant**(s)" of the mouth at a time.

◆ Subgingival irrigation—An antimicrobial solution is used to irrigate under the gums to further clean the area.

◆ Antibiotic treatment—Antibiotics are placed locally under the gums of any teeth that have pockets. The antibiotic is either delivered through a cord saturated with **doxycycline** (brand name Atridox) or in a gel (brand name Arrestin). The antibiotic is left in place and checked in approximately thirty days to evaluate the results.

◆ Nutritional supplements—The nutritional supplements calcium, vitamin C, antioxidants, and Coenzyme Q10 (mentioned earlier) can be taken to help enhance healing. (This is fully discussed in the next chapter.)

◆ Follow-up—The teeth are polished and you're told to return in about three to four months for evaluation and another professional cleaning.

Treatment for Moderate Periodontitis

The destruction of connective tissue attachments is more extensive with moderate periodontitis. The measurements around the teeth taken by the dentist may now read anywhere between four and six millimeters. Treatment for this stage will consist of any or all of the following. and may require several appointments:

◆ Repetition of treatments for mild periodontitis—Scaling and root planning, subgingival irrigation, antibiotics, nutritional supplements, and teeth polishing, as discussed in the treatment for mild periodontitis, are repeated.

◆ Additional antibiotics—If, after two to three months, there are areas still compromised and not improved, with pockets measuring over five or six millimeters, another round of local antibiotic therapy may be necessary. Oral antibiotics of very low dosage doxycycline (twenty-five milligrams) may also be prescribed for a few months.

♦ **Periodontal surgery**—The dentist may choose to refer you to a specialist (**periodontist**) for periodontal surgery to decrease the depth of the pockets.

♦ Follow-up—The gum disease may return after surgery if you don't follow proper home care and make regular dental visits.

Treatment for Advanced Periodontitis

At this point, the pocket depths indicating loss of attachment may well be more than six millimeters. Several or all of the teeth may be loose and may have to be extracted. Gum surgery along with the treatments listed previously may help save some of the teeth.

Gum Recession

Gum recession exposes the root surfaces of the teeth. This can pose some problems, such as tooth sensitivity, root cavities, and an unattractively long appearance of the affected teeth. The receded gums may appear red, swollen, and tender due to gum disease, trauma from aggressive brushing, or clenching and grinding the teeth.

Once the cause is identified, treatment should be followed as recommended by your dentist. If recession has caused a tooth to appear too long, the periodontist will **graft** tissue to make the tooth look normal. Tissue may be taken from the **palate** or some other area of the body to graft the gum.

Your Toothbrush

Another important factor to consider regarding healthy gum and bone is the cleanliness of your toothbrush. Would you eat all your

What happens in periodontal surgery?

The periodontist may perform flap surgery to thoroughly scale the entire length of the tooth and clean out infection. If you've lost considerable bone around any teeth, the periodontist may choose to **graft** bone into secure teeth in place. To encourage bone to grow back, the specialist may place tissue-stimulating proteins between the teeth and bone. This biocompatible material allows the bone to regenerate. For **bone graft**ing, the gums are flapped back surgically and all the teeth, including the root surfaces, are cleaned. Any irregular bone is smoothed and shaped. Artificial, synthetic, or natural (human donor) forms of bone may be used to rebuild vertical loss of bone. The area is covered with a bio-compatible membrane, which acts as a barrier to prevent down growth of the gums into the underlying bone. This membrane dissolves after several weeks. Stitches are placed, followed by another packing material to protect the tissue. There is usually discomfort and pain for a few days following gum surgery. Narcotic pain medication and antibiotics are prescribed.

food with one fork, rinse it with water, and then put it in the drawer to be used again at your next meal? That is basically what most people do with their toothbrush. Actually, it's worse because your toothbrush is usually kept in the bathroom and each time you flush your toilet, you're exposing your toothbrush to airborne bacteria. Studies have indicated that the bristles of the toothbrush harbor bacteria. In fact, if you use the same brush following a cold or flu, you can re-infect yourself and find it difficult to fight off a sore throat.

Soaking the bristles of a toothbrush in **hydrogen peroxide** and/or alcohol does not adequately destroy bacteria, although this helps. An antibacterial toothbrush purifier called "Purebrush" uses ultraviolet (UV) light to kill bacteria on your toothbrush. Research has shown that ultraviolet light is effective in eliminating micro-organisms. I highly recommend using this product as an important part of your home care, and suggest you use the unit to clean whatever sort of toothbrush you use, whether it's a power unit or manual type.

"An Ounce of Prevention is Worth a Pound of Cure"

This wise saying applies to all aspects of health. There should be no reason that people have to lose all or any of their teeth if they follow the recommendations in this book. Maintenance of healthy teeth and gums consists of two to four visits per year to the dentist for professional cleanings and evaluation, proper daily home care consisting of three-minute hygiene routines twice daily, and a healthy diet. When you weigh the difference between the costs (monetary, physical and emotional) and time it would take to treat advanced forms of gum disease against these relatively simple methods of prevention, the choice is obvious.

2

DIET AND NUTRITION

Beautiful Inside and Out

We are indeed much more than what we eat, but what we eat can
nevertheless help us to be much more than what we are.
—*Adelle Davis*

We've all heard our mothers tell us that if we eat too much
candy we'll get cavities. Until recent years, the relationship
between oral health and diet did not go much farther than the hazards of sugar. In May of 2000, the Surgeon General of the United
States issued a report on oral health. He stated that poor oral
health amounts to "a silent epidemic" promoting the onset of serious diseases such as diabetes, heart disease, and kidney disease—
which together are responsible for the deaths of millions of
Americans each year.

At its most basic level, as the saying goes, "we are what we eat,"
and poor oral health often begins with what we put in our mouth
as food. Our choices clearly aren't always wise. In fact, an estimated three out of four Americans suffer from gum disease—
a problem largely based on poor diet.

The results of many studies have helped the dental community understand that there is a strong link between oral health and balanced nutrition. Of course, balanced nutrition is the cornerstone
of health in general, but this is particularly true with fibromyalgia,

which is characterized by irritable bowel syndrome and many other conditions that may compromise the immune system. So it is especially important that people with fibromyalgia—whose immune systems are already compromised—eat well to build up their immune systems.

In the mouth, gum disease, cavities, and diseases of the tongue, **salivary glands** and soft tissues are infectious. Left untreated, they will persistently weaken the body's defense mechanism and its ability to combat other health conditions—including fibromyalgia.

Poor diet—one lacking adequate amounts of protein, vitamins, and other vital nutrients—not only contributes to lowered resistance to infectious conditions such as gum disease, but also undermines healthy development and growth of the body. Some long-term studies have established links between malnutrition and impaired skeletal growth, delayed tooth eruption, and abnormal growth patterns of the upper and lower jaw. Some of these traits can be passed on genetically for generations. For example, the need for orthodontic treatment to straighten teeth or treat TMJ may be seen with similar patterns in a family. Given such a familial pattern, poor nutrition is likely to aggravate these problems.

Eating Your Way to Healthy Teeth

One of the most common chronic human infections is periodontal, or gum, disease. As we discussed in the previous chapter, gum disease starts with inflammation and eventually leads to loss of bone that surrounds the teeth. Advanced gum disease causes loss of teeth. Along with gum disease, tooth **decay** is the other most common disease of modern civilization. If proper nutrients are not supplied to the body, it becomes impossible for the body to fight inflammation that leads to gum disease, infection and decay of tissues that lead to decay in teeth known as cavities.

I've already established that there is a link between oral health and systemic diseases such as diabetes, heart disease, and stroke.

Maintaining oral health will therefore reduce the risk of these diseases and help to minimize their effects. This is especially important news for people with fibromyalgia, whose health could be severely impacted if they contract any of these diseases. Certain nutrients are vital to promote healthy gums:

◆ Calcium and vitamin D are beneficial for healthy bone that supports and keeps your teeth in place.

◆ Antioxidants that include the vitamins A, C, and E are important for enhancing healing, maintaining tissue health, and reducing tissue destruction.

◆ Fish oils such as Omega 3-fatty acids help strengthen resistance to infection and tissue destruction.

◆ Selenium and zinc help reduce inflammation and promote healing.

◆ CoQ10 has been shown to be beneficial for repair of periodontal disease.

Stress and Poor Nutrition

Think of a "house of cards." Removing the good nutrition card at the base can make the whole assembly topple. Studies now indicate that poor nutrition can increase production and secretion of stress hormones (glucocorticoids) and lower the secretion of insulin, among other hormonal changes. Stress plays an important role in a variety of dental diseases. When people are under stress, they produce less saliva, which is very important for preventing tooth decay and gum disease. Poor diet also has affects the level of the same hormone glucocorticoids in the gums, so that gum tissue is unable to fight off inflammation. As a result, with chronic gum inflammation, the fatigue and general feeling of ill health due to your fibromyalgia become worse.

Stressed people tend to clench and gnash their teeth together by grinding them. In the next chapter I'll discuss why some people clench and grind their teeth while others don't. This can cause fractured teeth, receding gums, and TMJ. When we look at the whole picture, it all makes sense and becomes apparent that poor nutrition leads to a chain reaction of related problems:

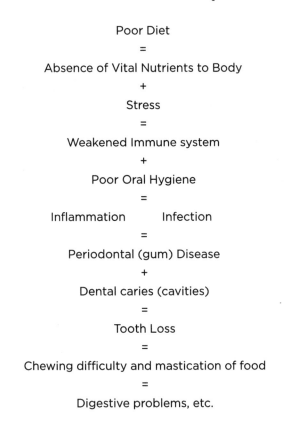

Poor Diet

=

Absence of Vital Nutrients to Body

+

Stress

=

Weakened Immune system

+

Poor Oral Hygiene

=

Inflammation   Infection

=

Periodontal (gum) Disease

+

Dental caries (cavities)

=

Tooth Loss

=

Chewing difficulty and mastication of food

=

Digestive problems, etc.

Poor Nutrition and Tooth Loss

Eating too little nutritious food and too much junk food is an inevitable route to cavities and tooth decay which will sooner or later require **root canal therapy** or tooth extractions. With a full set of teeth, the mouth is in equilibrium and food can be masticated (chewed) properly. With every removed tooth, an important component to chewing is lost, which negatively affects digestion of food. Digestion begins in the mouth as the saliva enzyme amylase breaks down starch to sugar. Missing teeth hamper this function and lead to changes in diet and eventually a poor nutritional state, further endangering your ability to cope with fibromyalgia.

Ill-fitting **denture**s also make it difficult to chew and break down food. Even with the best-fitting denture, chewing and tasting food is just not the same as with natural teeth. Many studies have shown that individuals with no teeth tend to eat foods higher in refined carbohydrates than non-dentures wearers. Their food may consist mostly of soft foods such as rice or mashed potatoes, with fewer vegetables that require more chewing. This diet may give rise to various systemic disorders.

Habitual use of alcohol, tobacco, and drugs, combined with a poor diet, tends to suppress appetite; people eat fewer nutrients than their bodies need, but continue to consume empty calories high in simple carbohydrates. Water is another very important component to dental health—it keeps the mouth moist and serves the body in innumerable ways without any ill effects. But people who drink soft drinks several times a day are exposing their teeth to high levels of acid. Consider the ingredients of colas: sugared carbonated water and phosphoric acid. Phosphoric acid is very corrosive. If a tooth is left in a bottle of cola, it has been reported to dissolve over time!

What exactly is the ideal diet for a healthy mouth? Even if we know what to eat to maintain proper nutrition, it's often hard to fit healthy meals into our busy schedules. Let's begin by looking at some useful facts about how certain foods affect fibromyalgia and oral health:

◆ Sugar. The higher the sugar content in foods, the greater the risk for tooth decay (cavities). A diet high in sugar for someone with fibromyalgia may aggravate irritable bowel syndrome and set off intestinal **candida** (yeast) infections.

The American Obesity Epidemic

The United States now has the dubious distinction of leading the world in obesity. This is no surprise, with fast-food restaurants on nearly every street serving high-fat, refined carbohydrate foods. People stop at these popular places for breakfast, lunch, and take their meals home to serve for dinner to the family. Not only are the foods served at most of these fast-food restaurants lacking in nutrition, the portions are often super-sized.

A report published in the July 2004 issue of *National Geographic* indicates portion sizes at fast-food restaurants have doubled since the 1970s. For example, a soda was eight ounces in the seventies. Today you are encouraged to purchase a thirty-two ounce soda—with French-fries thrown in for only a few cents more. The article reported that French-fry portions and the size of hamburgers have also doubled. Of course, soda refills are free. Adults and kids are staring in the face of serious health problems in the years to come, due to poor eating habits. Even school cafeterias have jumped on the bandwagon of fast foods and often sell soft drinks in vending machines. The fast-food industry has clearly scratched an itch in our busy lives. But while, in the short run, fast food may appear the easiest way to eat many meals, in the long term poor nutrition is likely to take a terrible toll.

◆ Refined carbohydrates. Eating foods high in starch increases the chance of developing cavities. A diet of highly refined carbohydrates in a person with fibromyalgia may also trigger onset of candida, aggravate irritable bowel syndrome, and cause weight gain. Most experts agree that limiting sugars and simple carbohydrates can help the person with fibromyalgia feel better. This is also true for many people who don't have fibromyalgia. Many people who are hypoglycemic or overweight are told to avoid sugar and refined carbohydrates, as are children with ADD (attention deficit disorder).

◆ Foods that ferment. A diet made up of sticky foods and fermenting foods such as breads and red meat can cause cavities. Once consumed, these foods ferment and convert to acid. Bacteria use the acid to destroy tissues.

◆ Acidic drinks. Frequently drinking fruit juices and soft drinks exposes the teeth to acids, causing tooth decay.

How to Achieve Proper Eating Habits

As with most worthwhile activities, it takes planning and discipline to change your eating habits. The following are simple steps to follow in order to reach your goal of eating right for oral health and a beautiful smile that will radiate from inside.

1. Make the decision that you are ready to make the change. Take a paper and pencil and take a long, honest look in the mirror. Do you need to make any changes to the way you look and feel? Jot them down on a "To Do" list. Are you overweight? Do you have bouts of irritable bowel syndrome due to certain foods that you know you shouldn't be eating, but can't resist? Psychological research suggests that it takes twenty-one days to change a behavior permanently, but you will start feeling a lot better immediately after you begin making the changes.

2. Plan what eating habits you need to change. This is easy when you're writing it down, so be honest. If you're stopping every day for a combo lunch that includes a giant soda, double burger, and fries, you know this is behavior that has to be changed. Foods can be very addicting, so the first step is admitting what is contributing to your situation and what you need to change and avoid in your daily routine.

3. Clean all the junk food out your cupboards and refrigerator and, after making your plan for your new eating habits, replace the junk with healthy foods from your list.

4. Make menus ahead of time for the whole week. You'll find this will make your life much easier and save time and money. Having to decide each day what's for dinner is a good excuse to stop at a fast-food takeout place.

5. Find a healthy eating program. There are many programs and guidelines available that help you decide what foods are healthy and what are not. Because everyone is different, it's a good idea to research which healthy eating program (or combination of programs) will work for you in meeting your specific goals.

The Glycemic Index

The glycemic index is a measuring system which evaluates and lists how much a particular food increases your blood sugar levels. Typically, foods that are carbohydrate-rich have higher GI numbers. For example, waffles have a GI value of 109, while peanuts are rated with a glycemic index of twenty-one. Studies have shown that the lower the GI of a food, the less the blood sugar level rises when it is eaten. Eating foods with high glycemic index values will raise the blood sugar level rapidly and you will feel hungry shortly after eating.

There are many popular diets such as Weight Watchers, Eat Right 4 Your Type, Fit for Life, and the Suzanne Somers's Diet. Several popular diets are discussed below, along with their value for people with fibromyalgia (see box). There should be no place for "Get Skinny Quick" diets that are not balanced. If you consume healthy, balanced food but less of it, you will lose weight and be healthy. A low carbohydrate diet is helpful to many individuals with fibromyalgia, because hypoglycemia is common with fibromyalgia. Dr. Paul St. Amand has excellent "strict and liberal" diets for Hypoglycemia on his web site: www.fibromyalgiatreatment.com. This type of diet—low in refined carbohydrates, low in fats and moderate in proteins—is also excellent for healthy teeth and gums.

The U.S.D.A. food guide pyramid recommends the following for a healthy, balanced diet:

- two to four servings of fruit
- three to five servings of vegetables
- six to eleven servings of breads and cereals
- two to three servings of meat
- two to three servings of milk products a day
- fats and sweets should be used sparingly

Many diet gurus feel this pyramid will work once you are healthy but, because many Americans have become overweight and unhealthy due to high carbohydrate diets, the USDA pyramid will have to be modified to meet the needs of a low carbohydrate diet.

Important Supplements for Healthy Teeth and Gums

Calcium:

Not only is calcium important for healthy teeth and bones, but it is also crucial for muscle contraction, nerve conduction, the beating of the heart, blood coagulation, glandular secretion, the production of energy, and the maintenance of immune function. In teeth and bone, calcium is found in the form of a calcium phosphate compound known as *hydroxyapatite*. Calcium is critical to people with fibromyalgia because of muscle related pain, risk of osteoporosis and its resulting effect on the jaw and teeth.

Calcium is found most abundantly in milk, yogurt, and cheese. Dark green, leafy vegetables such as collard greens, Chinese cabbage, mustard greens, broccoli, and bok choy are also high in calcium. Tofu, bones in canned sardines and salmon, orange juice, and soymilk also provide high amounts of calcium. Calcium is poorly absorbed from certain foods that are rich in oxalic acid (spinach, sweet potatoes, rhubarb and beans) and phytic acid, which is found in unleavened bread, raw beans, seeds, nuts, and grains. Vitamin D increases absorption of calcium and many supplements include it. Vitamin D is usually added to calcium supplements with a dosage of 100–400 IU/day.

I'm often asked which form of calcium is best for the health of teeth and gums. There are different types of calcium supplements available and its absorption depends on the type and how it is taken. Calcium supplements taken without food may increase the risk of kidney stones in women and possibly in men. Absorption tends to decrease with age, and especially in postmenopausal women, calcium levels tend to decline 0.21 percent per year.

Calcium carbonate should be taken with food in order for it to dissolve in the intestine and be absorbed into the blood. This is because this form of calcium requires an acidic environment to dissolve, and food provides that when stomach acids are present to digest food. On the other hand, calcium citrate does not require stomach acids to dissolve and should be taken on an empty stomach.

Most studies agree that calcium citrate is absorbed more efficiently than calcium carbonate. In one study, a 250-milligram dose of calcium citrate was found to be thirty-five percent absorbed, while the same 250-milligram dose of calcium carbonate was twenty-seven percent absorbed. Calcium absorption from milk was twenty-nine percent compared to the supplement. Calcium absorption increases when taken in doses of 500 milligrams or lower. Unabsorbed calcium is excreted in the feces.

Avoid dolomite, oyster shell, and bone meal forms of calcium supplements. These are naturally occurring calcium carbonate

Some Popular Diets

The Atkins Diet

Dr. Robert C. Atkins was the first to gain notoriety for developing a low carbohydrate diet. Keep in mind that this is more of a diet than a healthy nutrition plan. Usually, the purpose of a diet is to lose weight and may have to be modified once the weight loss goal is reached. A healthy nutrition plan will ultimately result in your ideal weight, but the purpose is not only to lose weight but also to develop healthy eating habits all the time. In fact, some "diets" may not be healthy at all, while all "healthy" nutrition plans are good for you. Critics of this diet say there isn't enough emphasis on bad vs. good carbohydrates, proteins and oils. The easy part of this diet is that there is no calorie counting or point system. His program consists of two phases:

- For fourteen days your food intake consists of not more than twenty to forty-five grams of carbohydrates per day, depending on your metabolic resistance. All forms of simple sugars and refined carbohydrates are eliminated. The twenty to forty-five grams of carbohydrates consist mostly of vegetables and some nuts.
- After fourteen days you move into a maintenance stage. In this stage, you will maintain your weight by not going over twenty-five to ninety grams of carbohydrates a day, depending on your metabolic resistance.

The Atkins diet is good for people with fibromyalgia because it emphasizes eliminating sugar and other simple carbohydrates. Since many of you do have dry mouth, eating foods that are high in sugar and carbohydrates will increase the risk of gum disease and tooth **decay**. The negative side is that eating large amounts of red meat may contribute to acid build up and tooth decay.

The South Beach Diet

The South Beach Diet consists of three phases. It does not encourage saturated fats, but encourages low fat foods.

- Phase one lasts two weeks and completely eliminates bread, rice, potatoes, pasta, fruit, candy, sugar, or baked goods. The only carbohydrates are the ones included in vegetables and salads. The claim is to loose up to thirteen pounds during this phase.
- Phase two introduces some more carbohydrates into the diet and has no time limit. You eat the food items on the list until you reach your desired weight.
- Phase three is the maintenance mode by which you continue to eat healthy, having changed your eating habits.

This diet is good for people with fibromyalgia because it emphasizes minimal amounts of simple carbohydrates. It also is more balanced than some other low carbohydrate diets such as the Atkins, since it recommends more variety of foods.

The Zone Diet

With the Zone Diet, a small amount of protein is combined with twice the amount of "favorable" carbohydrates. This is based on the theory that humans function most efficiently on a forty-thirty-thirty caloric ratio of carbohydrates to proteins to fat. This diet encourages high-fiber fruits, vegetables, beans, and grains.

This diet is good for people with fibromyalgia because it tends to be more balanced with types of foods to eat. It may take more planning since it is strict about the types and portions of food eaten.

Lindora Diet

The Lindora Diet is more regimented than the others, with daily weigh-in at a Lindora center and monitoring your urine with a ketone-measuring strip to determine if you are burning fat or carbohydrates (which means you're eating too many carbohydrates). You are also encouraged to weigh all portions of food.

This consists of two phases:

- Phase one is the Weight Loss/Metabolic Adjustment Phase and designed for a twenty-eight day module. During this phase, you limit your calories and carbohydrates intake, so that energy is obtained from fat stored in the body. The twenty-eight days are planned so that you alternate three days of "protein only" meals with three days of "weight loss menu" meals.
- Phase two involves fourteen days of metabolic adjustment. Days one and eight are protein only and the other days consist of metabolic adjustment menu meal.

This diet may be particularly difficult for people with fibromyalgia because of daily trips to the center and having to weigh portions of food. With all your fibromyalgia related physical challenges, this diet may be too taxing.

sources and may contain heavy metals such as lead, mercury, or arsenic. Calcium phosphate, calcium lactate, and calcium gluconate should not be taken, since they contain only a very small percentage of elemental calcium in each supplement.

There are interactions between certain drugs and calcium that you should be aware of if you are taking any of the following:

Biphosphonates (sometimes used for osteoporosis or bone fractures)—absorption is decreased if taken with calcium.

Quinolones and tetracycline (antibiotic)—absorption is decreased if taken with calcium.

Levothyroxine (used for hypothyroidism)—absorption may decrease when taken with calcium carbonate.

Estrogen—increases production of vitamin D and therefore helps increase calcium absorption.

Tannins in tea—binds calcium in the intestine and decrease its absorption.

Magnesium and phosphorous— also require vitamin D for absorption and decrease calcium absorption if taken excessively by decreasing the vitamin D available to aid calcium absorption. Recommended daily intake of phosphorus is 3,000 to 4,000 and 350 milligrams of magnesium.

The National Osteoporosis Foundation suggests 1,500 milligrams of calcium is needed per day for postmenopausal women not taking estrogen and adults sixty-five years or older. The recommendation is not to take more than 2,500 milligrams of calcium per day. Constipation, developing calcium kidney stones, and possibility inhibiting absorption of iron and zinc from food are some results of calcium toxicity.

Antioxidants:
Antioxidants are substances produced by the body that slow cellular "oxidation," which contributes to aging and to certain diseases. Antioxidants fight "free radicals." These free radical molecules can cause damage to biological molecules associated with aging, strokes, and a number of other diseases, with some evidence pointing to a role in fibromyalgia. Vitamins C, A, E, and CoQ10 are antioxidants. Antioxidants are critical to people who have fibromyalgia because of action against free radicals. If you are

living with fibromyalgia, you need all the help you can to help fight damage to cells, and antioxidants are a good place to start.

Vitamin C—or ascorbic acid—is a water-soluble vitamin important not only for healthy teeth and gums, but also for wound healing and strengthening blood vessel walls. Deficiency in vitamin C will result in swollen, bleeding gums and eventually loss of teeth through advanced periodontal disease. Vitamin C can be found in many foods including most fresh fruits and vegetables such as citrus fruits, green vegetables, tomatoes, and berries.

Vitamin C supplements often contain *bioflavonoids*. These are not vitamins but compounds derived from lemons, oranges, and grapefruits. It is believed that flavonoids work to enhance the effects of vitamin C. Rose hip vitamin C is another form of supplement. The rose hip is the swollen ovary of the flower, which produces seed after the petals of a blossom falls. Once the petals fall off, the only part that remains of the rose is the "rose hip." Rose hips are the major source of natural vitamin C. They also contain flavonoids. If you suffer from the chronic dry mouth or burning mouth as a result of your fibromyalgia, vitamin C will be most helpful in helping to repair tissue and help prevent breakdown of gum tissue.

Vitamin A is a fat-soluble vitamin and is important for bone growth and the surface lining (mucous membrane) of the mouth, and night vision. Vitamin A should be an important supplement to take if as a result of your fibromyalgia you have dry mouth or burning mouth. Foods that are rich in vitamin A include carrots, apricots, sweet potatoes, spinach, squash, and cantaloupes. Other foods rich in vitamin A include beef and chicken liver. Excessive amounts of vitamin A (over 10,000 IU), on the other hand, may lead to bone loss and increased hip fractures. High amounts of vitamin A used for prolonged periods may affect the mouth with bleeding gums, dry mouth, and dry, cracked lips. This vitamin is supplied in two forms. Beta-carotene is the form to use and retinol is the kind to avoid. The beta-carotene form is a stronger antioxidant and is found mostly in vegetables and fruit sources. Retinol is found more in meat organs and cod liver oil. Retinol has found popularity in skin creams as an anti-aging ingredient.

Vitamin E is important for function of muscles and nerves. Like all antioxidants, it fights naturally occurring substances that may damage cells in the body called "free radicals." Excellent sources of vitamin E are wheat germ and vegetable oils. Vitamin E is supplied naturally or synthetically and comes in the form of: d-alpha, d-gamma, d-delta, and d-beta-tocopherol. Some studies suggest a mixture of all of these types is the best form of vitamin E to take. The natural form is normally known as d-alpha-tocopherol, while the synthetic vitamin E is called dl-alpha-tocopherol. This vitamin is important if you have fibromyalgia since it can help with muscle pain as well as with TMJ, or if you tend to require numerous root canals due to nerve damage.

The Food and Nutrition Board of the National Academy of Sciences has established the RDA in milligrams for vitamin E, taking into account only alpha-tocopherol. However, most supplements are labeled in internationals units (IU). To convert IU of synthetic vitamin E into milligrams, multiply the IU listed on the label by 0.45, (for example 33 IU x 0.45 = 15 mg). To convert natural vitamin E to milligrams, you must multiply the IU by 0.67 (for example 22 IU x 0.67 = 15 mg).

CoQ10, also known as ubiquinone or coenzyme Q10, is an antioxidant that was discovered in 1957 by researchers at the University of Wisconsin. CoQ10 is found in every cell in the body and plays an important role in the energy producing parts of the cell, called mitochondria. This natural substance stimulates the use of oxygen at the cellular level. Most of the research on CoQ10 has been done in Japan. Some studies indicate this is useful in the management of periodontal disease. Most of the harmful bacteria that cause gum disease thrive most when there is lack of oxygen. Because CoQ10 improves the use of oxygen at the cellular level, it makes sense that it might be helpful with gum disease as well as improving the overall fatigue of fibromyalgia.

A recommended daily allowance has not been established for this substance since the body can manufacture it on its own. However, a typical recommended dose for gum disease is thirty to one hundred milligrams daily, divided into two to three doses.

R.D.A. (recommended daily allowance) is the amount of vitamins and minerals set in the United States, needed by healthy individuals. This amount may vary depending on the age, sex, and physical condition of the person.

R.D.A. REQUIREMENTS:

Supplement	Vitamin C	Vitamin A	Vitamin E	CoQ10
Adults—male	50–60 mg	3000 IU	10–15 mg	Not established
Adults—female	50–60 mg	2333 IU	8–15 mg	Not established
Pregnant females	70 mg	2500 IU	15 mg	Not established
Breastfeeding	90–95 mg	4000 IU	19 mg	Not established
Smokers	100 mg	4000 IU	19 mg	Not established
Children 4–10	25 mg	400 IU	6 –7 mg	Not established
Children under 3	20 mg	375 IU	5–6 mg	Not established

There is no doubt that proper nutrition maintains the health of the whole body, including not only the teeth but also the supporting structures of the teeth. We live in a time where we have a multitude of dietary choices that will affect our health and well-being. Fundamentally, the choice comes to a diet consisting of large amounts of unhealthy processed foods full of fat, sugars and bleached white flour or healthy, correctly proportioned, balanced meals consisting of protein, vegetables, fruits, and whole grains. In terms of our dental health and appearance, if we consider how we hope to appear in the future, either with a healthy beautiful smile with our own teeth, or with removable plastic dentures, our dietary choices and menus will be obvious.

Healthy snacks for healthy mouths

- Celery with cheese or a tablespoon of peanut butter
- Vegetables such as cucumbers, zucchini, and broccoli. (Try with dip made of non-fat yogurt and/or low fat sour cream seasoned with garlic powder, and your favorite seasoning. Also good with low fat blue cheese or ranch dressing.)
- Fruit
- Rice cakes
- Frozen fruit bars with no added sugar
- Unbuttered popcorn
- Low or non-fat yogurt
- Low or non-fat cheeses
- A few nuts
- Homemade smoothie (Make with your favorite fresh fruits including banana and low- or non-fat milk or soymilk.)
- Hard-boiled egg

If you have fibromyalgia, these foods may prove particularly helpful in your diet because they are low in simple carbohydrates, but balanced with healthy choices of fruit, vegetables, and protein.

3

TMJ

Treat the Jaw Joint and Cure Your Headache

As with fibromyalgia, for many years people who complained of a similar set of symptoms, which we now call temporomandibuluar joint disorder (TMJ), were told it was all in their head. They were either sent for therapy or given tranquilizers, pain medications, and antidepressants for life. Fortunately, we now recognize TMJ, like fibromyalgia, as a very real, diagnosable disorder. Other terms that describe this condition include myofascial pain dysfunction (MPD), craniomandibular dysfunction (CMD), or the acronym TMD. So as not to cause confusion, in this chapter it will be referred to as TMJ.

Fibromyalgia and TMJ have many similarities. Some of the common symptoms in both include:

◆ Poor concentration
◆ Headaches
◆ Dizziness
◆ Sinus problems with post-nasal drip or nasal congestion

- Ringing in the ear (**tinnitus**)
- Neck and shoulder pain with trigger points

Even some of the causes that result in symptoms for both TMJ and fibromyalgia are similar, such as trauma, nutritional deficiencies, hormonal changes, anxiety, and stress. A very common symptom shared by the two is the manifestation of trigger points. A trigger point is an area in a muscle that is painful when touched or pressed. These areas feel like knots, which restrict blood flow in the area. When biopsies from these areas were analyzed, they were found to contain high levels of lactic acid, hyaluronic acid (which contributes to swelling), carbonic acid (a mild acid), and **serotonin**, which is a vasoconstrictor. Trigger points illicit pain, muscle spasms, fatigue, numbness, and weakness. Pain can occur just where pressure is applied, but can sometimes also affect distant areas, a phenomenon called "referred pain." With TMJ, the trigger points are usually in the neck, shoulder, and back areas. Another similarity between fibromyalgia and TMJ is that both commonly occur in women between the ages of twenty and fifty, peaking during reproductive years. Not all individuals with TMJ have been diagnosed with fibromyalgia; however, most people who have fibromyalgia usually also have TMJ.

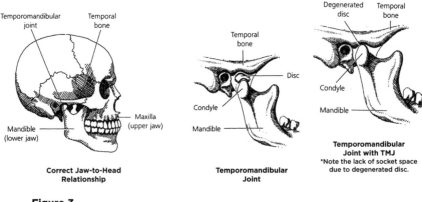

Correct Jaw-to-Head Relationship

Temporomandibular Joint

Temporomandibular Joint with TMJ
*Note the lack of socket space due to degenerated disc.

Figure 3

How Do I Know If I Have TMJ?

There are many distinct symptoms that are associated with TMJ. Not all the following symptoms are always present, but as the disorder progresses, most will appear at some time or another. These include:

- Clicking, popping, ringing noises in the ear
- Headaches
- Pain and pressure behind the eyes
- Jaw pain
- Pain in neck area
- Problems with jaw movement during eating or yawning
- Lockjaw and limitations in opening and closing the jaw properly
- Sinus problems
- Pain on chewing, especially hard foods
- Problems with the bite

By placing your fingers directly in front of the ears and slowly opening and closing your mouth, you will feel the movement of the jaw and the jaw joints. If you hear any noises when you do this, or feel any pain, you may have signs of TMJ.

If you suspect that you grind or clench your teeth, or have had braces (orthodontic treatment) in the past, ask your dentist to examine you to determine if you have TMJ. If you have normal range of motion when you open and close your mouth, you should be able to place three fingers in your mouth between your upper and lower teeth while your mouth is open, and feel no pain. If you can only fit one or two fingers in your mouth, then you have limited range of motion and should consult your dentist for treatment.

What If My Jaw Makes Noises When I Eat?

Under normal conditions, the jaw's temporomandibular joint makes two kinds of movements. When the mouth is opened slightly, a *hinge-like* movement is utilized. When the mouth is opened very wide, the jaw *slides* forward and down and does not use the hinge unit. Closing the jaw follows this pattern in reverse.

The jaw joint consists of a socket, which is part of the skull and is located in front of the ear and a ball (condyle), which is part of the **mandible** (lower jaw). When the mouth is closed, the condyle sits in the socket cushioned by a cartilage called an "articular disc." This disc allows a smooth transition of the jaw from a resting position to the initial opening with the hinge movement.

If the jaw joints are not functioning properly and smoothly, you will hear noises as the condyle changes from a hinge position to the sliding movement. The noises are either called **crepitus** (crunching or grinding noises) or **tinnitus** (ringing in the ears). Crepitus or **crepitation** is brought about when there is contact between hard tissues (bone against bone). This occurs when there is either damage to the articular disc or to the ligaments that help it function so that there is no longer a cushion between the condyle and the socket, causing bone to hit against bone. This bone-against-bone movement produces grinding or grating noises.

In another instance of crepitus, the articular disc sticks in an improper position and fails to move smoothly with the condyle when the jaw is opened, temporarily locking or dislocating the jaw. Jiggling or moving the jaw back and forth with quick movements causes the disc to be released from its improper position and allows it to catch up with the condyle so the two move together again. As the disc attempts to unlock and catch up with the condyle, you hear the popping noise.

Tinnitus, or ringing in the ear, is often associated with TMJ, as well. It results when the condyle is displaced into the rear of its socket, exerting pressure on the inner ear and causing a loss of balance and hearing. Besides TMJ, there are other causes for tinnitus, such as medications, sinus infections, or wax build-up in the ear canal. However, jaw misalignment due to misaligned jaw joints or muscles can also bring about this annoying ringing in the ears.

What Should I Do If I Think I Have TMJ?

Treatment of TMJ is a multidisciplinary job. Start with a dentist who is trained to treat TMJ. Eventually you must see either a physical therapist or chiropractor, as well. Because other structures of the head can cause symptoms similar to those experienced with TMJ, a consultation with an otolaryngologist (ENT specialist) is also needed to rule out problems with the ear and sinus.

As with any other health condition, it's very important to determine the cause of TMJ for proper treatment. The following are some of the common causes:

♦ Trauma to the head and neck (auto accidents, etc.).
♦ Habits such as **clenching** or grinding the teeth; chewing ice; biting nails or pencils.
♦ Stress (which may bring about habits such as clenching or grinding the teeth).
♦ Misalignment of the jaw due to heredity.
♦ Poor bite due to missing teeth, poorly made fillings, **crowns**, or dentures.
♦ Poor posture, including not only how you stand or sit, but also carrying heavy bags or holding the telephone receiver between your shoulder and ear for long periods of time while talking. This places stress on the muscles of the head and neck, leading to misalignment.

TMJ involves problems with the musculoskeletal system of the head, neck, shoulders, and back. Once the cause of symptoms is determined, management is important or the symptoms will recur, as they often do with disorders involving the musculoskeletal system. The following are treatment options based on severity of symptoms:

Self Help

If you've been suffering from chronic TMJ pain, it's possible you've become resolved that this is just the way things will be for the rest of your life. This need not be so. Millions of people have found ways to reduce and control pain. The more your knowledge and confidence grow, the more you will take responsibility for your health and life. When illness affects your body, muster up all your mental resources to overcome the situation. Don't undermine yourself by crying the blues—instead, get ready to take charge. You have a battle to win! You will notice that the more you learn, practice and keep your chin up with a positive attitude, the better you will be able to overcome pain. Start by asking yourself:

- What am I usually doing when the pain is worse?
- What am I doing when pain is least noticeable?
- When did I first notice the pain?

These are important data to gather in considering your situation. If you wake up in the morning in pain, that could mean you were grinding or clenching your teeth during the night. If eating is painful, there could be functional problems. The next action step would be to find a dentist and a team of other health care practitioners trained in this field who can help determine the cause and what to do about it. This takes research and determination. I don't advise going from one practitioner to another looking for "pain cures," but do your homework, find the qualified team and start treatment.

Below is a list of things you can do to help with your TMJ symptoms:

- At bedtime, take a hot shower or bath. This helps tense muscles to relax, helping you to sleep better, and perhaps will help with clenching or grinding if that is a nighttime habit.

◆ Do some simple stretching exercises for the neck and back, as prescribed by your physical therapist or chiropractor. This may also help relieve tension build up in that area and promote relaxation.

◆ Apply moist heat or ice.

1. Heat increases circulation, decreases joint stiffness, pain, and muscle spasm. It's mostly helpful in chronic situations. It can be applied via a washcloth heated under hot water in the sink, cooled to a comfortable temperature, applied to the area for a few minutes and repeated. Make sure to check the temperature before applying it, to prevent burns.

2. Cold application is indicated for acute pain to help relieve muscle spasm, myofascial traumatic pain, or acute inflammation. Use either an ice bag or cold pack.

3. Try both cold and heat and use whichever helps give relief.

◆ **Biofeedback** is a method of using your body's information to modify behavior. Everyone practices some form of biofeedback. For example, when you see a scary movie, your heart may race. You would be applying biofeedback if you were to watch the same movie, but learn to not allow it to affect your emotions to the point where it makes your heart beat fast. This method may not work for everyone. Biofeedback can be a useful tool, but one that requires practice and demands personal responsibility. It's rather like using the scale to supply information about your weight; the information is only useful if you are willing to modify your food intake if you weigh too much or too little. A professional can provide you with specialized biofeedback equipment to help you understand your body and your control of it, or you can practice the technique at home.

The best use of biofeedback for TMJ is to learn to do mental and emotional relaxation exercises that will relax the muscles in the jaw. Stress is a major contributor to muscle tension and pain and their effects on the jaw joint. It's best to practice biofeedback on yourself before you feel pain or before a stressful situation comes up. This way, when it actually does occur, you're ready to handle it and not allow it to cause damage. Of course, this is easier said than done, and does take practice. One method to practice biofeedback on yourself is the following: Find a nice, quiet area to sit or lie down. Read a book or favorite passage from a book which you know gives you hope and overall good feelings. My favorite passages that uplift me every time I read them are the Book of Psalms in the Bible. You may have other books, poems or passages that uplift you. Meditate on them and let them overcome feelings of helplessness or hopelessness. This takes diligence and must be practiced daily, or every time you begin to feel hopeless, stressful, or anxious.

♦ Laughter is always good medicine and sometimes the best. Rent funny videos to watch, read the comics in your local newspaper, and laugh heartily when in the mood.

♦ When you have jaw pain for an extended period, you have to treat the jaw as if you have had a sprained ankle and are told not to walk on that ankle. Because the mouth has so many uses, such as speech, yawning, and eating, it's difficult to give it a good rest. Here are a few ways to keep from overusing the jaw:

1. Don't yawn too widely.
2. Eat soft foods if your jaw is painful. Avoid hard foods (crunchy French bread, pizzas, or carrots).
3. Don't talk with the telephone held between your neck and shoulder.
4. Don't carry heavy purses or other items.
5. Don't wear high heels.
6. Practice good posture while standing or sitting.
7. Take regular breaks and stretch if you use a computer often.
8. Remember that massages may be helpful.

Dental Therapy

Typical treatment methods for TMJ that your dentist can perform include surgical and non-surgical approaches. The non-surgical is the more common approach.

♦ Orthotic **splint** or **mouthguard**. This non-surgical treatment involves a bite plate called an orthotic splint (mouthguard) made by a dentist and worn during the night and, sometimes, all day. The dentist takes an **impression** of either the top or bottom jaw or both and usually fashions the splint from clear acrylic. The splint repositions the jaw to its normal alignment, moving the jaw down and forward and relieving the pressure caused by the misalignment. Usually, within a week or so, patients feel some relief and less pain. If you hear ringing in your ears or other noises, the orthotic splint should help. However, at some point if damage is too severe, the noises may not go away. For the orthotic (splint) to succeed in managing the symptoms, other factors must be addressed, such as proper posture, stress management, physical therapy, and elimination of harmful habits.

♦ Medication. The dentist may recommend injection of **local anesthetic** or steroids in the joint space to bring relief. Medications such as muscle relaxants, anti-inflammatory, or pain management drugs may also be prescribed.

♦ Surgery. If the problem is not with the muscles that move the jaw but with the joint itself, then surgery may be needed. If the damage is minor, such as a damaged cartilage, a small instrument called an arthroscope is used as a telescope for the surgeon to see inside the joint and make repairs as needed. If the damage is more severe, then a procedure called **arthroplasty** is performed. The surgery may involve recontouring the bone of the jaw joint, or artificial replacement of the disc in the joint.

Physical Therapy

◆ Dr. Janet Travell's technique of spray & stretch, usually performed by a physical therapist or chiropractor. Dr. Travell, the physician who treated former President Kennedy, developed this technique for relieving muscle pain. A glass or metal bottle with a calibrated nozzle containing either ethyl chloride or another substance called fluori-methane is sprayed on painful muscles. This results in a momentarily chilling effect of the area. This allows the muscle to relax and it is then gently stretched and brought to the normal resting length. The technique provides temporary relief from pain and cramps.

◆ Transcutaneous electrical nerve stimulator (TENS) or **ultra-sound** to help relax muscles. With the TENS unit, electrodes usually contained in pads are placed over painful muscles. Small electrical impulses are sent to nerve fibers to block pain signals. Ultra-sound uses high frequency sound vibrations (above the range we can hear) through a machine. Gel is applied to the skin to help the sound waves travel through the area. The metal wand or "head" of the ultra-sound machine is moved in small circles to help bring relief to painful muscles.

◆ Specific TMJ exercises recommended by osteopath, chiropractor, or physical therapist.

Other forms of therapy:

◆ Stress management.
◆ Nutritional counseling.
◆ Psychological counseling.
◆ **Acupuncture**, shown in studies to temporarily relieve pain.

Is There a Cure?

Most people have found that, like fibromyalgia, TMJ demands management of symptoms for most of their life or understanding and minimizing the triggers that bring on the symptoms. Once the pain is under control, you will notice very quickly what events cause pain and symptoms to resurface. By paying attention to your body, you will learn to avoid certain actions that normally bring on pain. Examples of likely pain triggers include sitting in front of a computer for a long period without stretching, talking on the phone while holding the phone between your neck and shoulder, or chewing hard food on only one side of your mouth.

Make a list of the things you do that may contribute to your jaw disorder. Next to each item on the list, write ways to remind yourself to correct or avoid that behavior. If you listen to your body and take responsibility for preventive action, you will not suffer pain from TMJ, and may even notice relief from headaches.

4

FIBROMYALGIA AND GUAIFENESIN

What's All the Fuss about Salicylates?

Although no cure has been found for fibromyalgia, a variety of methods to manage its symptoms have been suggested. Because fibromyalgia affects so many functions in the body, prescription drugs, exercise, and nutrition have all been presented as treatment options.

There are many symptoms associated with fibromyalgia that have already been discussed in detail. They include: fatigue, musculoskeletal pain with trigger points, problems with concentration and memory, insomnia, depression, headache, TMJ, irritable bowel syndrome, dry eyes and mouth, and tingling in the extremities (see Introduction, page xviii).

Paul St. Amand, MD, an assistant clinical professor at UCLA's Department of Endocrinology and author of the foreword to this book, found an interesting correlation between dental tartar and gout medication that led him to form a theory about what may cause fibromyalgia and how to manage the symptoms. In his book, *What Your Doctor May Not Tell You About Fibromyalgia* (coauthored by Claudia Marek), Dr. St. Amand noted that when **guaifenesin**, an expectorant that thins mucus, was taken in specific doses, symptoms associated with fibromyalgia such as pain and fatigue were diminished, with the person eventually becoming asymptomatic. He believes that the mechanism for this treatment is tied to the energy-producing actions of cells within the body of a person who has fibromyalgia. Due to phosphate retention within the cell's mitochondria (the parts of the cell that produce of energy), the cells are not able to generate enough energy. He argues that guaifenesin helps stop the excess phosphate build-up in cells by causing the kidneys to release it.

A Word about Dr. St. Amand's Guaifenesin Protocol

Treatment of FMS symptoms with the supplement guaifenesin was initially developed by Dr. Paul St. Amand. At the present time this protocol is not generally recognized by the medical community and is still in the theory stage. One double-blind study on FMS and guaifenesin therapy was performed at the University of Oregon in 1995 and concluded that the effects of guaifenesin are similar to a placebo (a substance such as a sugar pill, used in clinical trials to compare effects of a particular treatment versus no treatment). Dr. St. Amand does not agree with the findings because the study was flawed in many aspects. It only utilized twenty subjects, used only one dosage of guaifenesin, and did not restrict the use of salicylates, which are said to block the effects of the supplement. Further studies are being planned to prove the effects of guaifenesin on symptoms associated with fibromyalgia.

There is just one catch to this protocol: patients must avoid all topically applied substances (applied to the skin or surface tissues of the body) that contain ingredients called salicylates. Salicylates block the effect of guaifenesin by competing for the renal tubule sites on which guaifenesin acts to release the phosphate. Salicylates, or salicylate acid, are produced naturally in many plants and herbs. Salicylates have been used for more than a hundred years in the form of aspirin (acetylsalicylic acid) to treat inflammation, pain, and fever. Salicylate use in people who are especially sensitive or allergic may cause asthma, tinnitus (ringing in the ears), and vertigo. These compounds are sometimes added to products such as oils, lotions, and over-the-counter medications.

Many people with fibromyalgia have tried the **guaifenesin protocol** and found it successful in the management of their symptoms. The numbers of people using this protocol is growing every day, as support groups and web sites are spreading throughout the nation and the world with positive testimonies. However, many people avoid the protocol when presented with the thought of using only salicylate-free products. It takes discipline and time to go to the store and read every label. Even if a product was found to be salicylate-free and purchased previously, it may not be salicylate-free the next time you buy it, because ingredients in products are frequently altered. Many products don't have to list all of their inactive ingredients, which make the situation even more difficult. To make life easier, the back of this book lists names of companies that only sell salicylate-free products. As the number of people on the guaifenesin protocol increases, so will the choices and availability of salicylate-free products. Below are listings of all salicylate-free, over-the-counter dental products and those normally used at the dental office.

Salicylate Free Over-The-Counter Dental Products

Toothpaste:
Grace FibroSmile (888) 883-4276
Tom's of Maine has a variety of "low salicylate" toothpaste but it contains sodium lauryl sulfate, which I do not endorse. This is a harsh industrial detergent and used as such.

Fluoride Gel

Home Care (888-883-4276)
Colgate Gel-Kam Fluoride Treatment
Available through prescription only
Colgate Prevident 5000 Prescription Dental Cream (fruit)
Dinosaur Fluoride (Bubble gum flavor) (800-245-1825)
Phos-Flur Anti-Cavity Fluoride Rinse

Mouthwash

Grace FibroSmile, all flavors
Plax Original Flavor Rinse
Sav-On Pre-Brushing Anti-Plaque Dental Rinse
Chlorhexidine gluconate, antimicrobial mouth rinse prescribed for gum disease.
Compounded by and available through Mulberry Pharmacy in Florida. Your dentist must fax a prescription to them.
New Sweet Breath Sorbet Lemon Flavored Breath Spray
Oxyfresh Oxygene "Unflavored" Mouthrinse

Chewing Gum

Grace FibroSmile

Dry Mouth Moisturizer

Salivart

Denture Adhesives

Fixodent Original Cream
Fixodent Free Cream Ingredients
(Avoid Fixodent Fresh Cream Adhesive and Fixodent Powder Adhesive because they contain peppermint oil.)
Secure Denture Cream

Denture Cleaners

Secure by Den Tek available at 888-883-4276

Breath Sprays
Grace FibroSmile

Teeth **Whitening**
Crest Whitestrips
Opalescence TresWhite Melon Flavor

Salicylate Free Products Used by Your Dentist

Whitening
All Opalescence Melon Flavor
Zone (one-hour whitening)
   Available in dental offices; ask for the unflavored.

Dental Polishing
The dentist or hygienist usually uses mint polishing paste. The other flavor that is available to them is cherry, but even that may contain mint. Instead of taking a chance, when you go for a routine dental cleaning, take a tube of Grace FibroSmile toothpaste (see above) with you for the polishing part of your professional cleaning.

Impression Materials
Many are available that do not contain mint or salicylates. Tell your dentist that you need to use one without mint flavor.

Permanent Cements
Many are available that do not contain mint or salicylates. Tell your dentist that you need to use one with without mint flavor.

5

MEDICATIONS AND THE MOUTH

Managing Those Side Effects

This chapter will focus on which medications or supplements may adversely affect the mouth and what to do about it. All the possible medications prescribed for fibromyalgia are listed in this chapter, along with their affects on the mouth. If you have any of the symptoms associated with the medications, make sure you discuss the matter with your physician and seek alternative medications. If you have to take the medication and there are no alternative choices, your dentist can help minimize dental problems arising from these side effects.

Physicians often prescribe medications for the many symptoms that characterize fibromyalgia. These prescription and over-the-counter drugs may include those for pain, depression, muscle relaxants, allergies, and sleep disorders, just to name a few. Most physicians are more concerned with treating specific symptoms and tend to be less concerned with the side effects these drugs may have on the mouth. In fact, many physicians don't appear to consider this effect at all. However, medications are often taken for long periods of time, especially if they are effective in providing relief for the symptoms. Eventually, some adverse changes may begin to be noticed in the mouth, including dry mouth, abnormal gum growth, and tooth discoloration.

In order to treat any dental disease, as in any other part of the body, identifying the real cause from among many possibilities leads to the appropriate treatment. Dry mouth, abnormal gum growth, and tooth discoloration could be caused by factors other than the side effects of drugs. Use of alcohol-containing mouth-wash, salivary gland conditions, smoking, anxiety, stress, radiation therapy, and drug abuse may cause dry mouth.

Abnormal gum growth may be due to gum disease, pregnancy (known as pregnancy tumor), sensitivity to toothpaste or mouth-wash, and deficiencies of vitamin C or other nutrients. Tooth discoloration can be caused by developmental abnormalities (including genetics); exposure to certain substances (such as coffee, tea, colas, tobacco); cavities; malnutrition and nutritional deficiencies; trauma, bleeding disorders, and infections.

Sometimes one side effect of a particular medication may give rise to other problems. For example, dry mouth may cause discoloration of teeth. One of the functions of saliva is to remove food and debris (plaque) from the tooth and in-between the teeth. As food and plaque remain on the teeth, black stains will eventually form.

Medications That List Dry Mouth as a Side Effect

Many drugs, including those listed below, decrease the amount of saliva secreted in the mouth. Saliva serves many purposes in the mouth. Not only does it lubricate and help with breakdown and digestion of food, but it also has a buffering effect on acids in the mouth and helps remove food and plaque from the teeth. With abnormally low salivary flow, there is an increased risk for cavities and gum disease. Saliva is also important for denture wearers because it helps keep the denture in place and more comfortable.

If you notice that your dry mouth seems drier than normal when you begin taking any of the medications on this list, ask your physician if an alternate medication might be available. If this is not an option, then consider the following steps to prevent more severe dental problems:

- ◆ Use over-the-counter saliva substitutes such as Salivart.
- ◆ Brush and floss twice a day.
- ◆ Use chewing gum containing **xylitol**.
- ◆ Drink plenty of water
  (Sip it frequently during the day and keep it at bedside at night.)
- ◆ Avoid alcohol and caffeine.
- ◆ Don't smoke.
- ◆ Avoid spicy foods.
- ◆ Avoid citrus and acidic juices such as orange, grapefruit, lemon, and tomato.

Medications That May Cause Dry Mouth

ANOREXIANT
Adipex-P, Fastin, Ionamin, Zantryl (phentermine)
Anorex SR, Adipost, Bontril PDM (phendimetrazine)
Mazanor, Sanorex (phendimetrazine)
Pondimin, Fen-Phen (fenfluramine)
Tenuate, Tepanil, Ten-Tab (diethylpropion)

ANTI-ACNE
Accutane (isotretinoin)

ANTIANXIETY
Atarax, Vistaril (hydroxyzine)
Ativan (lorazepam)
Centrax (prazepam)

Equanil, Miltown (meprobamate)
Librium (chlordiazepoxide)
Paxipam (halazepam)
Serax (oxazepam)
Valium (diazepam)
Xanax (alprazolam)

ANTICHOLINERGIC/ANTISPASMODIC
Anaspaz (hyoscyamine)
Atropisol, Sal-Tropine (atropine)
Banthine (methantheline)
Bellergal (belladonna alkaloids)
Bentyl (dicyclomine)
Daricon (oxyphencyclimine)
Ditropan (oxybutynin)
Donnatal, Kinesed (hyoscyamine with atropine, phenobarbital, scopolamine)
Librax (chlordiazepoxide with clidinium)
Pamine (methscopolamine)
Pro-Banthine (propantheline)
Transderm-Scop (scopolamine)

ANTICONVULSANT
Felbatol (felbamate)
Lamictal (lamotrigine)
Neurontin (gabapentin)
Tegretol (carbamazepine)

ANTIDEPRESSANT
Anafranil (clomipramine)
Asendin (amoxapine)
Elavil (amitryptaline)
Luvox (fluvoxamine)
Norpramin (desipramine)
Prozac (fluoxetine)
Sinequan (doxepin)

Tofranil (imipramine)
Wellbutrin (bupropion)

ANTIDIARRHEAL
Imodium AD (loperamide)
Lomotil (diphenoxylate with atropine)
Motofen (difenoxin with atropine)

ANTIHISTAMINE
Actifed (triprolidine with pseudoephedrine)
Benadryl (iphenhydramine)
Chlor-Trimeton (chlorpheniramine)
Claritin (loratadine)
Dimetane (brompheniramine)
Dimetapp (brompheniramine with phenylpropanolamine)
Hismanal (astemizole)
Phenergan (promethazine)
Pyribenzamine (PBZ) (tripelennamine)
Seldane (terfenadine)

ANTIHYPERTENSIVE
Capoten (captopril)
Catapres (clonidine)
Coreg (carvedilol)
Ismelin (guanethidine)
Minipress (prazosin)
Serpasil (reserpine)
Wytensin (guanabenz)

ANTI-INFLAMMATORY ANALGESIC
Dolobid (diflunisal)
Feldene (piroxicam)
Motrin, Advil (ibuprofen)
Nalfon (fenoprofen)
Naprosyn (naproxen)

ANTINAUSEANT/ANTIEMETIC
Antivert (meclizine)
Dramamine (dyphenhydramine)
Marezine (cyclizine)

ANTIPARKINSONIAN
Akineton (biperiden)
Artane (trihexyphenidyl)
Cogentin (benztropine mesylate)
Larodopa (levodopa)
Sinemet (carbidopa with levodopa)

ANTIPSYCHOTIC
Clozaril (clozapine)
Compazine (prochlorperazine)
Eskalith (lithium)
Haldol (haloperidol)
Mellaril (thioridazine)
Navane (thiothixene)
Orap (pimozide)
Sparine (promazine)
Stelazine (trifluoperazine)
Thorazine (chlorpromazine)

BRONCHODILATOR
Atrovent (ipratropium)
Isuprel (isoproterenol)
Proventil, Ventolin (albuterol)

DECONGESTANT
Ornade (phenylpropanolamine with chlorpheniramine)
Sudafed (pseudoephedrine)

DIURETIC

Diuril (chlorothiazide)
Dyazide, Maxzide (triamterine and hydrochlorothiazide)
HydroDIURIL, Esidrix (hydrochlorothiazide)
Hygroton (chlorthalidone)
Lasix (furosemide)
Midamor (amiloride)

MUSCLE RELAXANT

Flexeril (cyclobenzaprine)
Lioresal (baclofen)
Norflex, Disipal (orphenadrine)

NARCOTIC ANALGESIC

Demerol (meperidine)
MS Contin (morphine)

SEDATIVE

Dalmane (flurazepam)
Halcion (triazolam)
Restoril (temazepam)

Medications That May Cause Overgrowth of Gum Tissue

With overgrowth of gum tissue (**gingival hyperplasia**), the gums appear swollen. Hormonal changes, medications, and certain diseases such as leukemia can cause overgrowth of gum tissue. However, plaque remains the most common culprit, complicated by other factors, such as specific drugs. When the cause is a result of the side effects of certain prescription drugs, surgery may be the only course of action. However, even though the possibility of overgrowth exists with some of these medications, meticulous daily home care and regular professional cleanings may prevent or diminish the effects of the overgrowth.

The area most often affected is the upper anterior (front) gum area. With long-term use of problematic medications, the overgrowth becomes severe and the gums around all the teeth become swollen. The **gingiva** will appear pink and spongy with especially pronounced areas between the teeth. The condition is painless, but may push the teeth apart as the gums continue to grow. If not treated, the gingiva may grow to cover the entire tooth. To prevent this from happening, practice proper home care before the medication is taken.

The following medications can result in gingival hyperplasia:

- Dilantin, Kapseals (Phenytoin)—used for Parkinson's and to control seizures.
- Nifedipine—used for treatment of high blood pressure.
- Cyclosporin—an immunosuppressant used to prevent rejection of organ transplants.

Medications That May Cause Gum Sores or Discolorations

Certain medications may result in tooth discoloration, sores, and inflammation of the gums. These include chemotherapeutic agents used for cancer therapy and oral contraceptives. Your dentist will recommend more frequent check-ups (at least every three months) and certain anti-microbial rinses to help counteract these side effects. However, some of the anti-microbial rinses are themselves known to cause staining. Gum sores and staining may result from taking:

- Anticholinergics.
- Antihypertensives.
- Antipsychotics.

- Antihistimines.
- Chlorhexidine Rinse (0.12 percent), stains teeth with long-term use.
- Cetylpyridinium chloride in certain mouthwashes.
- Iron solutions used for iron-deficient anemia, may cause black stains.
- **Stannous fluoride**, may turn teeth brown.
- Tetracycline, stains teeth when taken while either primary (baby) or permanent (adult) teeth are developing. This happens whether the pregnant mother or the child takes the tetracycline during the development stages of the teeth. Once the teeth have developed, this antibiotic does not discolor teeth.
- Minocycline, an antibiotic similar to tetracycline and prescribed for acne, may stain the teeth green or blue-gray with long-term use.
- **Doxycycline**, an antibiotic used for gum disease, is typically taken in low doses for a long period of time.
- **Fluoride** taken in excess during the formation of the teeth may cause **fluorosis** of the teeth, causing the teeth to appear chalky or to have streaks of white lines on the enamel. For adults, cosmetic dentistry, usually with **veneer**s or crowns, can improve the appearance of these teeth.

Medications That May Cause Bleeding

Anticoagulants are commonly used to help reduce blood clotting. These include heparin and warfarin, used for treatment of heart disease and stroke. Aspirin also has anticoagulant properties. Among people who use these medications, it may be difficult to control bleeding following a tooth extraction, periodontal (gum) surgery, or other procedures that may result in bleeding. Your physician may recommend discontinuing the medication for a few weeks before dental surgery.

Drug Abuse and Its Dental Effects

Approximately seven to ten million Americans suffer from the effects of fibromyalgia. Some may become addicted to the medications they use to control their symptoms, such as Vicodin (a pain medication), Ambien (a sedative), anti-anxiety medications, or others. Addiction to any drug causes emotional as well as physical breakdown. Abuse of prescription drugs may bring about dry mouth and neglect of routine dental home care. Illegal drugs can also cause oral problems. Marijuana use stains the teeth and stimulates plaque buildup, leading to gum disease. Cocaine rubbed on the teeth will result in gum line cavities.

If you are about to start taking a medication, ask your physician if any side effects may influence the health of the mouth. If you're aware that a particular medication may cause a problem in the mouth, see your dentist as soon as possible for an evaluation. With regular professional cleanings and check-ups by your dentist, problems with your teeth and gums can be avoided, prevented or treated while still minor. If these problems go untreated, a domino effect may occur, with side effects turning into major, costly problems. Dry mouth can give rise to gum disease. This in turn can increase the risk of heart disease, stroke and last but not least, loss of teeth.

In many cases, discontinuing a drug allows the dental side effects to abate. However, if cavities or gum disease are present, they must be treated. If problems have resulted from a medication, your dentist can help. Treatment may range from routine three- to six-month check-ups and cleanings to cosmetic dentistry such as whitening the teeth. Please don't neglect necessary treatment because doing so will not only adversely affect your mouth but may also worsen your fibromyalgia symptoms by placing added stress on the immune system.

6

SNORING AND SLEEP APNEA

Opening the Airways for a Restful Night

As you very likely know, most people living with fibromyalgia fail to get a good night's sleep. With poor quality sleep or sleep deprivation, even a person without fibromyalgia will begin to feel many of the symptoms that fibromyalgia patients endure. Headaches, fatigue, depression, mood swings, irritability, sleepiness during the day, and lack of concentration are some of the symptoms associated with lack of sleep that anyone who has fibromyalgia knows well.

Studies have determined that most individuals with fibromyalgia do not experience **delta sleep** (stages three and four of non-REM sleep), which is important for the body's ability to restore and rejuvenate. Most of the time they only reach what's called **alpha activity**, which is a state of light sleep. There is no clear explanation for this. We do know that common to both fibromyalgia and sleep disturbances are depression and widespread pain in the body.

There are many classifications of sleep disorders. In this chapter we'll concentrate on sleep-related breathing disorders (SRBD), because this is an area that your dentist can help with. This type of sleep disorder is very common and includes:

- ◆ **Snoring**
- ◆ Obstructive **sleep apnea** (OSA)
- ◆ **Hypopnea**
- ◆ Sleep **bruxism**

Snoring

Snoring affects about fifty percent of men and twenty-five percent of women at some time or another, and mostly affects people over the age of forty. Although snoring can be very annoying and can cause married couples to seek separate bedrooms, it can also be a signal of a serious medical condition. When there is an obstruction in the back of the throat and the airway collapses, airflow causes loose tissue in the area to vibrate, making the harsh snoring sound. As a person falls asleep, the **soft palate** (roof of the mouth), tongue and throat relax. The **uvula** is a hanging piece of tissue at the end of the soft palate and the entrance to the throat. As airflow exerts more pressure to enter the narrowed and collapsed airway, the uvula vibrates, making the snoring sound.

Snoring is common in overweight individuals, especially those with much fatty tissue in the neck area. Weight loss can reduce snoring, if that is a contributing cause. Avoiding alcohol before retiring also helps. Sleeping on your side versus lying on your back may also help reduce snoring. Lying on your back naturally makes the tongue rest toward the back of the throat, closing the airway.

There are several options for the treatment of snoring:

- **Surgery**—Excess tissue is trimmed surgically from the entrance to the airway. This is a painful procedure and requires an overnight stay at the hospital with a few days of recovery time. The procedure is irreversible and may not be totally effective.
- **Continuous positive airway pressure** (CPAP)—A pressurized mask is worn tightly over the nose while you sleep. Air is forced through the mask via a hose attached to a small generator pump at your bedside. This device eliminates snoring in most cases and prevents sleep apnea, but it limits movement during sleep and may cause drying of the nose and throat. While this method is widely used, it is uncomfortable and difficult to use when traveling.
- **Somnoplasty**—This is a type of surgery that is also called radio-frequency tissue volume reduction. A low-intensity radio-frequency signal is used to remove part of the soft palate. This does not require a hospital stay and requires only local anesthesia. This technique is fairly new and more data about its effectiveness is being gathered.
- **Laser surgery**—This another treatment for light snorers in which the surgeon uses a laser to remove the uvula. It is also performed in an outpatient setting with local anesthesia. Repeated surgeries (up to five) may be needed, performed four to six weeks apart.
- **Dental oral devices** or appliances—These can be very effective for reducing snoring and opening the airway. Many physicians and patients are unaware that these devices exist. They come in a variety of shapes and types, and vary in cost from $300 to $600. Some common brands include Norad, Therasnore, Silencer Custom, and Silent Nite. Most dentists provide these kinds of devices. The dentist takes a mold of your teeth and sends it to a laboratory for fabrication. You return to the dentist to pick up the device, along with instructions on how to use it.

Obstructive Sleep Apnea

Obstructive sleep apnea (OSA) occurs when breathing stops for ten seconds or longer several times during sleep. The word apnea is Greek-derived and means "without breath." Due to this constant interruption of sleep, the person wakes up with a headache, is fatigued and irritable, an usually very sleepy during the day. Snoring and sleep apnea frequently go together.

Like snoring, apnea arises from an obstruction of the airway. The collapsed airway causes a momentary halt in breathing, which lessens oxygen flow to the blood. As your brain recognizes this change, it awakens you to resume breathing. At times, you may awaken gasping for air and feeling as though you are choking, while at other times you may not even remember awakening. This constant interruption to sleep (sometimes ten or more times an hour) will cause impaired sleep which denies the body and mind the rest they need.

Several factors can cause increased risk of sleep apnea:

◆ Enlarged tonsils.
◆ Heredity (sleep apnea sometimes runs in families).
◆ Use of excessive alcohol at bedtime.
◆ Lying on your back instead of your side.
◆ Being overweight, especially in the neck area.

Sleep apnea and **hypopnea** are similar except that with sleep apnea, breathing during sleep totally stops for ten seconds or longer, while in hypopnea breathing decreases for ten seconds or longer. The episodes may repeat more than 100 times during the time of sleep.

In many communities there are sleep clinics that can evaluate the extent of your sleep disorder. An overnight sleep study called a **polysomnogram** can determine the presence and severity of OSA. Treatment options for sleep apnea include surgery to remove tonsils and adenoids or to correct a deviated nasal septum or your dentist can help with a specific device. In extreme cases where the sleep apnea is life threatening, a surgical procedure called a "tracheostomy" is performed. A small opening is made in the patient's neck and a metal or plastic tube is placed in it. During the day the opening is covered, but at night it is opened to allow air to pass through without blockage. Other forms of surgery are also sometimes performed to remove excess tissue blocking the airway. Repositioning the jaw surgically can open the airway as well.

Sleep bruxism is usually referred to as **bruxism** or grinding of the teeth and is often related to stress. Bruxism is a common symptom of fibromyalgia, and can further complicate the oral issues that so frequently occur in fibromyalgia (discussed in Chapter Three on TMJ).

Recent studies have demonstrated that bruxism occurs mainly during "Stage II Sleep" (the non-rapid eye movement phase) and during "REM sleep" (the rapid eye movement phase). Neither of these stages is the deepest periods of sleep. The American Academy of Sleep Medicine (AASM) describes bruxism not as a disorder, but as an activity that disrupts sleep. Sleep bruxism may occur, along with sleep apnea and snoring.

In some individuals, bruxism can be as loud and annoying as snoring, with gnashing of the teeth making a very loud and distinct sound. However, bruxism can also be very silent with the person not aware of it at all. Many times the dentist will ask patients who have signs of grinding or clenching the teeth if they are aware of doing it, and the majority are not. If you grind your teeth your dentist usually sees specific patterns of wear on the teeth. The tops of chewing (occlusal) surfaces are either hollowed out or flattened. The tips of the front teeth (incisal edges) may be flattened from the constant wear. Another common observation is receded gums due to the heavy pressure and force brought about by the grinding and clenching. It's been estimated that the human jaw is capable of 900 pounds of pressure during bruxism.

With continued clenching and grinding, the teeth can become sensitive and fracture. Another by-product is stress on the jaw joints causing temporomandibular joint disorder (TMJ), which is common with fibromyalgia.

A simple mouthguard or one of the dental oral devices for sleep apnea or snoring will go a long way toward stopping the harmful effects of bruxism. Teeth that may have been damaged due to the wear will have to be treated. With fibromyalgia patients, the appliance may have to be used on and off for the rest of their lives.

Snoring and sleep apnea can be not only annoying, but also dangerous to one's health. Learn about your treatment options, consult with your physician and dentist, and seek treatment to help you sleep more soundly and restfully. Remember, restful sleep is an important ally in your efforts to deal with the effects of fibromyalgia on your life.

7

DRY MOUTH

Moisturizing Relief for the Mouth

One of the most frequent symptoms of fibromyalgia—and one that's mentioned extensively throughout this book—is **dry mouth**. Like so many symptoms related to fibromyalgia, dry mouth presents something of a chicken and egg quandary. Which causes which? Does fibromyalgia cause dry mouth or, in some cases, does dry mouth bring on symptoms of fibromyalgia? We can't yet answer that question with certainty, but we are sure that dry mouth is an almost universal complaint in fibromyalgia and that it can lead to a whole host of other issues, including dental problems, gum disease, bad breath, **burning mouth syndrome** and many internal organic disorders. This chapter will review some of the information available about mouth dryness and offer you some techniques to help you cope with this troubling issue.

Dry mouth can have devastating effects. It can make swallowing and talking difficult, can make the teeth prone to cavities, and result in gum disease. Having dry mouth once in a while is not abnormal, especially if you're anxious, under stress or very thirsty. But if your mouth feels dry most or all of the time, this could be a symptom of certain diseases, including fibromyalgia, or a side effect of certain medications or conditions. A normal, healthy adult produces approximately three pints, or forty-eight ounces, of saliva per day. Saliva serves very important functions besides keeping the mouth moist and helping us seal envelopes. Dry mouth or **xerostomia** is a by-product and symptom of salivary glands that are not producing adequate amounts of **saliva**. When your mouth feels dry, you are obviously not producing adequate amounts of saliva.

Three pairs of glands secrete saliva. The *parotid* gland produces a watery secretion, and is located in the cheek area above the **molars**. The *submaxillary* glands produce a mixed watery and mucous-like secretion and are located under the lower jaw near the molars. Lastly, the *sublingual* glands secrete a thicker mucous and can be found under the tongue.

How much and what type of saliva we secrete is regulated by the autonomic nervous system (ANS) which also regulates all reflexes and involuntary actions, such as muscle reflexes and the action of glands. In other words, we really don't have much control over how much or what type of saliva we produce and dry mouth is mostly a side effect of other situations in our body.

As an aside, some stimuli can trigger our brains to increase salivation. These signals include the sight, aroma or thoughts of certain foods. For example, just the thought of squeezing a lemon into your mouth, or the smell of bacon cooking in the morning, may stimulate the salivary glands. We tend to take for granted that saliva always keeps our mouths moist until our mouth becomes so dry that we have difficulty eating certain foods, such as crackers. To better understand the importance of saliva, let's take a closer look at its functions.

- ◆ Saliva lubricates and binds food, making it easier to swallow.
- ◆ Saliva promotes tasting of food.
- ◆ Saliva helps with talking.
- ◆ Saliva contains the enzyme "amylase," which initiates the digestion of starch into maltose.

♦ Saliva contains the enzyme "lyozyme" which helps neutralize bacteria in the mouth. When the mouth is moist, this enzyme flushes out food debris and keeps the mouth relatively clean.

♦ Saliva helps keep breath, teeth and gums healthy. During sleep, saliva flow is reduced considerably, often resulting in "dragon breath" or "morning breath." Individuals with dry mouth are more prone to cavities and gum disease.

Persistent dry mouth increases the incidence of dental decay and other oral health problems. Because of a chronically dry mouth, the sense of taste is diminished, chewing and swallowing are more difficult, gum disease, and Burning Mouth Syndrome (BMS), (see Chapter Four), are more likely to develop. It has been reported by the Academy of General Dentistry that more than one million adults in the United States, mostly post-menopausal women, are affected by burning mouth syndrome. As this persists, changes in eating habits, irritability, depression, and reduced desire to interact with others are all likely to result.

Some of the symptoms that accompany dry mouth or xerostomia, may include:

♦ Bad breath
♦ Difficulty tasting food
♦ Increased plaque, tooth decay and gum disease
♦ Dry lips, with cracks in the corners
♦ Difficulty swallowing
♦ Difficulty talking
♦ Burning sensation of the tongue

Dry Mouth Can Have Many Causes

Numerous factors and health conditions can cause and contribute to dry mouth. Sometimes blood tests or other diagnostic means may be needed to identify the cause. The following are some of the common contributors to dry mouth:

- Fibromyalgia and **Chronic Fatigue Syndrome**
  These conditions can cause dry mouth mostly due to medications.
- HIV/AIDS.
- Diabetes.
- **Sjorgren's Syndrome.**
- Radiation therapy for cancer.
  Radiation can cause total or partial loss of saliva, making it extremely difficult to eat, and adversely affect the teeth.
- Chemotherapy
  Chemotherapy can thicken saliva, causing the mouth to feel dry.
- Tobacco
  Excessive pipe, cigar, cigarette smoking, or chewing tobacco will result in dry mouth.
- Alcohol
  Heavy alcohol consumption can result in dry mouth, and eventually lead to cancer of the mouth.
- Stress and depression
- Autoimmune diseases such as rheumatoid arthritis
- Mouth breathing due to blocked nasal passages
- Menopause and hormonal changes
- Aging

Additionally, there are approximately 400 medications that may cause dry mouth. See pages 55–59 for a list of many of them.

Medications appear to be the most common cause of dry mouth. If dry mouth is severe and causes problems with chewing and swallowing, and you are taking medications in the categories above, ask your physician for dosage modifications, or substitutes.

Treatment Options

In order to permanently cure dry mouth, the cause must be determined. If the cause is a medication, the dosage or prescription should be changed. If there is a problem with the salivary glands, your doctor can prescribe medicine to make them work properly. In the meantime, there are ways to restore moisture while you are determining the cause of the dry mouth. The treatment for dry mouth and burning mouth syndrome are similar.

Treatment must begin with a thorough professional dental visit for cleaning and, if needed, gum treatment and repair of decay in teeth. Proper home care is essential in preventing decay and gum disease because saliva is not present in adequate amounts to impede the presence of harmful bacteria. Several products and activities can help control dry mouth:

- Using oral care products such as Biotene that contain enzymes to lubricate the mouth.
- Brushing and flossing twice a day.
- Using over-the-counter saliva substitutes such as Salivart.
- Chewing gum containing xylitol.
- Sucking on hard candy sweetened with xylitol.
- Drinking plenty of water, sipping it all day and during the night.
- Avoiding alcohol and caffeine.
- Avoiding tobacco products.
- Avoiding spicy foods.
- Avoiding juices high in acid such as orange, grapefruit, lemon, and tomato.
  (These promote an acidic oral environment, making you prone to increased tooth decay and gum disease.)
- Breathing through your nose, instead of your mouth.
  (Seek treatment if you have blocked nasal passages.)

- ◆ Visiting the dentist regularly to prevent decay and advanced gum disease due to dry mouth.
- ◆ Using a humidifier in your room to add moisture.*

*Note: Make sure you don't overuse this. An overly moist environment encourages growth of mold or dust mites.

8

BAD BREATH

Does a Dragon Live Inside Your Mouth?

Getting ahead in a difficult profession requires avid faith
in yourself. That is why some people with mediocre talent,
but with great inner drive, go much further than people
with vastly superior talent.
—*Sophia Loren (1934–)*

know you have your plate full with all the symptoms and
problems fibromyalgia causes. Sorry, but add one more—bad
breath.

You can't have faith and confidence in yourself if you have
bad breath. To put it mildly, it's very embarrassing to realize you
have bad breath when you're having a conversation with someone. This is such a social taboo it's even difficult to tell someone
they have bad breath. It's a sure way to make self-confidence
evaporate. We realize how negative bad breath is when we are
engaging in a conversation with someone who has **halitosis**
(bad breath) and notice how downright offensive it is. Many sur-
veys indicate this is something most people worry about at some
time or another, especially if they are speaking to a special someone or wake up with morning bad breath with their loved ones
close by.

How to Tell If You Have Bad Breath

There are a few simple steps to determine if you have bad breath:

1. The easiest way is a battery operated palm held instrument called "Breath Alert." As you breathe into it, it gives a reading within seconds of odor: none, mild, or strong.
2. Ask loved ones to tell you. Sometimes those close to you may not tell you unless you ask because it might hurt your feelings.
3. Cupping your hand and smelling it is not very effective.

Also, take inventory of your dental health. Below are some questions to ask yourself to determine whether you have bad breath:

◆ Do you practice good daily oral hygiene?
◆ Do you keep regular, three- to six-month dental visits?
◆ Do you drink enough water?
◆ Do you smoke?
◆ Do you have a bad taste in your mouth?
◆ Do you avoid snacking on junk foods?
◆ Does your mouth usually feel dry?
◆ Do you wear old dentures that are ill-fitting, chipped or cracked?
◆ Do people step back or turn their face from you while you're speaking to them?

If the answer to these questions is "yes," then the likelihood is strong that you have bad breath. Unfortunately, bad breath is likely to be a problem for you because of your fibromyalgia. As you know only too well, fibromyalgia causes many problems, from intense pain, to depression, and general fatigue. Often medications are prescribed to help manage these symptoms. A side effect of many of these medications is dry mouth, which brings on bad breath. Dry mouth can also be a sign of gum disease. We now realize that, besides the bad breath it causes, gum disease can be life-threatening because, as many studies have shown, it increases the risk of heart disease and stroke.

Dry mouth isn't the only cause of bad breath, of course. We all know that such foods as onions and garlic cause offensive odor from the mouth. However, foods contribute only about fifteen percent of the causes of bad breath. They result in temporary bad breath that disappears when the offending food is not eaten. The other eighty-five percent of halitosis originates in the mouth and involves bacteria.

There is one underlying factor that brings about the actual malodor from the mouth: **anaerobic sulfur producing bacteria** (*fusobacterium, actinomyces*). The word anaerobic means "without oxygen." In other words, these bacteria like environments that are devoid of oxygen. In ideal conditions there is a balance between the anaerobic and aerobic bacteria that are present in the mouth to maintain health. However, under certain conditions, when the balance is tilted to the **anaerobic bacteria**, they proliferate.

The anaerobic bacteria digest protein in foods and the by-products they release are sulfur-producing gases, which we perceive as bad breath. Foods rich in protein (such as meats, fish, cheese and other dairy products) are more likely to bring about bad breath because they cause the breakdown and release of more by-products from the bacteria. Meat contains the amino acids cysteine and methionine, which are rich in sulfur. Coffee, whether it is caffeinated or not, contains high levels of acid. Any liquid or food high in acid helps anaerobic bacteria reproduce. It is not unusual to have bad breath while having a cup of coffee. When bacteria come into contact with sulfur producing foods, sulfur compounds are released. These are called "volatile sulfur compounds" or VSCs—resulting in halitosis.

Since these bacteria don't like oxygen, they form colonies in areas that are hidden and difficult to clean. These areas include the back of the tongue and under the gums. Unless these two areas are meticulously cleaned daily, bad breath will be present.

Many activities and conditions can cause bad breath, some perhaps surprising. These causes include:

- **Medical conditions.** Bad breath can be caused by conditions such as diabetes mellitus (acetone-like smell); fasting; kidney failure (fishy odor); liver disease; embolic disorders; and gastrointestinal reflux disease, in which stomach acids back up into the esophagus and even the mouth.
- **Allergies, Sinusitis.** Allergies are often accompanied by nasal and sinus fluid buildup. Bacteria can grow in this stagnant fluid and result in bad breath.
- **Post-Nasal Drip.** If **sinusitis** is not treated, it becomes chronic, resulting in drainage from the infected sinus down the back of the throat, known as post-nasal drip. Post-nasal drip allows mucous to drain onto the back of the tongue and throat. The bacteria in that area break down the mucous, releasing sulfur gases. If you take antihistamines to decrease the drainage, that brings about dry mouth, which as we know, promotes more malodor.
- **Snoring.** Most snoring is due to blocked airway. This produces dry mouth, a common cause of bad breath.
- **Smoking and Tobacco Products.** Because tobacco products produce a dry and unhealthy oral environment, bad breath and tobacco go hand-in-hand.
- **Poor Dental Care, Oral Hygiene, and Bad Breath.** Lack of regular dental treatment can contribute to bad breath. Old, corroded silver fillings, fractured fillings, ill-fitting crowns and dentures can all result in bad breath because any rough areas offer good places for bacteria to accumulate and multiply. When your dentist suggests replacing an old filling or crown, it's a good idea to do so. If dental treatment is ignored, a problem could develop into an abscess and eventually, a foul-smelling and foul-tasting discharge may be released through the gums (gum boil).

Regular professional cleanings are another very important factor in keeping the mouth healthy and keeping bad breath at bay. Professional cleanings every three to six months will help clean hard-to-reach areas and guard against deterioration of oral tissues. If there's an unaddressed dental problem, it will not go away on its own. Breath mints or mouthwash might mask the problem temporarily, but will do nothing to solve it.

◆ **Dry Mouth.** Dry mouth is common with fibromyalgia and often results from medications taken for variety of symptoms such as depression and anti-anxiety. Common over-the-counter medications, especially antihistamines, also cause dry mouth, as do mouthwashes that contain alcohol. Other causes include drinking excessive amounts of soft drinks and alcoholic beverages. Saliva has a buffering affect against acids in the mouth and is rich in oxygen. With dry mouth there is less saliva and less oxygen, which is the type of environment in which sulfur-producing bacteria tend to thrive. As these anaerobic bacteria multiply, they produce more sulfur as a by-product and therefore malodor.

Dry mouth promotes the development and growth of plaque (the thin film upon which bacteria build and accumulate) because the inner layer of plaque contains no oxygen and allows the growth of these sulfur-producing bacteria. The back of the tongue is an area that is especially rich in anaerobic bacteria. This area is generally ignored and not cleaned. It also contains deep grooves along with a thick coating, which again makes it the ideal environment for bacterial growth. It is this back part of the tongue from which much bad breath emanates.

◆ **Poor Diet.** If your diet consists mostly of fast foods high in fat, and simple carbohydrates high in sugar, then you are not promoting a healthy body and mouth. As a result, the immune system is less able to combat the production of bacteria that result in gum disease, of which bad breath is a by-product. Fasting and dieting also cause bad breath.

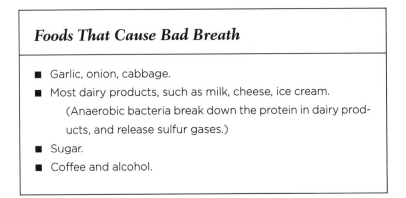

Foods That Cause Bad Breath

- Garlic, onion, cabbage.
- Most dairy products, such as milk, cheese, ice cream. (Anaerobic bacteria break down the protein in dairy products, and release sulfur gases.)
- Sugar.
- Coffee and alcohol.

The good news is that bad breath can be eliminated. Because your condition predisposes you to bad breath, the last thing you need to do is compound the problem. So here are some things to consider that help tame the dragon in your mouth.

First let's put together important components of what you'll need to begin:

1. A soft manual or power toothbrush. Don't get a toothbrush with a brush head that's too big for hard-to-reach areas such as the back molars. The handle should fit comfortably in your hand.

2. Toothpaste that does not contain sodium lauryl sulfate. With those on the guaifenesin protocol (this involves taking a particular supplement for treatment of fibromyalgia and is discussed in chapter 17), the toothpaste must be salicylate free. Toothpaste that contains baking soda and a tartar control ingredient such as pyrophosphate is best. If you have sensitive teeth, potassium nitrate is the active ingredient that will help. I also don't recommend toothpaste that contains

artificial sweeteners such as saccharine. Xylitol is preferred over other sweeteners because it also helps prevent tooth decay.

3. Floss, either waxed for normal teeth. You'll need tape if you have spaces between your teeth. You'll need a floss threader if you a **bridge** in your mouth. (A bridge contains a false cap to replacing a missing tooth, and is attached to adjacent teeth on either side of the missing tooth. The only way to clean this area is with a floss threader).

4. A tongue cleaner. These come in a variety of shapes and materials. Some are plastic loops, while others are metal or plastic handles with scrapers at the end. They usually come with instructions, but the concept is to clean the tongue by gently scraping over the surface of the entire tongue. You can also clean your tongue with your toothbrush.

5. Mouthwash with no alcohol. Preferable mouthwashes contain baking soda and use only xylitol as a sweetener.

Six Steps to End Bad Breath

Now let's take these steps:

1. Every morning and evening, brush each side of every tooth very thoroughly. This should take a good two to three minutes.

2. Clean your tongue, especially the back. You can use either a toothbrush or a tongue cleaner, described above. If need be, hold your tongue with tissue while you clean the back area, where the bad breath bacteria hide and cause most of the damage. If you tend to gag, take a deep breath and slowly count to four while you're cleaning the tongue. The more you concentrate on cleaning this area, the more successful you'll be in combating bad breath. For more about tongue cleaners, see Chapter Thirteen.

3. Rinse with mouthwash (non-alcoholic), swishing it around as long as you can stand it.
4. In between meals, rinse with water and chew gum sweetened with xylitol, which stimulates saliva flow to help clean the mouth.
5. Drink plenty of water.
6. Floss at bedtime.

You should notice immediate results after following these steps. If after a week of diligence, you still have bad breath, see your dentist. The problem may be gum disease or dental problems that require some sort of professional treatment.

You can eliminate bad breath despite your fibromyalgia. Follow the steps outlined in this chapter and you'll be surprised how easy it is. But tackling bad breath does require a commitment and a routine. Brush carefully. Floss often and thoroughly. Clean the back of the tongue. Seek routine dental treatment. Oh, and don't blame your toothpaste or mouthwash. Unfortunately, some people have done just that and switch from brand to brand or make their own toothpaste with baking soda and/or hydrogen peroxide or use hydrogen peroxide as a mouth rinse. This can be very hazardous to the mouth. Baking soda on its own is abrasive and hydrogen peroxide is unpredictable and can cause tissue damage if used for long periods of time. Keep the harmful bacteria at bay on a daily basis with thorough yet gentle cleaning that will destroy bad breath for good.

9

BURNING MOUTH

Cool Off for Relief

First keep the peace within yourself, then you can also
bring peace to others.
—*Thomas a Kempis (1380–1471)*

It can be very difficult to be at peace when your mouth feels like
it's on fire. When most people talk about burning mouth, the
cause was likely a piece of pizza right out of the oven, a steaming cup
of coffee, or hot bowl of soup. The mouths of people with **burning
mouth syndrome (BMS)** also feel as if they're burning, but the
sensation never goes away. Research indicates that this is yet
another problem common among people living with fibromyalgia.

Like fibromyalgia, TMJ, Epstein Barr, and chronic fatigue syndrome, burning mouth syndrome was at one time considered to
arise from the emotional problems of menopausal women. Now we
know that burning mouth syndrome typically appears in women
approximately three years before and up to twelve years after
menopause. Although burning mouth syndrome sometimes affects
adolescents and adults of both sexes, it is especially common in
women. According to the Academy of General Dentistry, up to one
million American adults may currently suffer from some degree of
burning mouth syndrome.

What Is Burning Mouth Syndrome?

The most common complaint among individuals with burning mouth syndrome is a sensation similar to burning the mouth with hot coffee. Burning mouth syndrome, or "glossodynia," means "tongue pain." The pain and burning can involve the lips, tongue, the roof of the mouth, the inside of the cheeks and the back of the mouth or throat. Another term used to describe this condition is "stomatodynia" or mouth pain. The symptoms appear suddenly and without any warning and may never go away except during sleep. The pain has been usually reported to diminish during eating or drinking. It tends to increase as the day goes on and reaches a peak by late afternoon to late evening. The discomfort can range from moderate to severe, and has been compared to toothache pain. The level of discomfort can vary from day to day. However, in many individuals it can sometimes interfere with falling asleep, causing symptoms associated with sleep disturbances, such as irritability, anxiety, or depression. With these individuals, burning mouth contributes to lack of sleep and also often creates a bitter taste in the mouth.

The problem with burning mouth syndrome is that there are no clinical and laboratory findings that provide a definitive diagnosis or tell us much about it physiologically. Burning mouth syndrome is diagnosed after ruling out yeast infection in the mouth, vitamin deficiencies, and diabetes. However, certain conditions are usually present with burning mouth syndrome, and these help to distinguish it from other disorders:

◆ Dry mouth.
   Many people with burning mouth syndrome complain of dry mouth, although the condition doesn't seem linked with problems affecting the salivary glands or with decreased saliva flow.
◆ Taste alterations, including a metallic taste and loss of bitter taste in the mouth.

♦ Difficulty swallowing, other throat problems.
♦ Chronic anxiety or depression.

There don't seem to be any particular factors that precipitate the symptoms, although burning mouth syndrome most commonly appears in women right before and after menopause. Approximately one-third of patients relate the time of onset to a dental procedure, recent illness, or medication course. Once the symptoms begin, burning mouth syndrome often continues for several years, often running its course at about six to seven years and then either diminishing in symptoms or disappearing.

Causes of Burning Mouth Syndrome

The causes of burning mouth syndrome remain uncertain, but could be simply a reaction to a food or medical product or to multiple factors. The following are some of the possible causes for burning mouth syndrome:

♦ Ill-fitting dentures, which over time can cause changes in the soft tissue under the plate, resulting in disease (lichen planus, candidiasis) that causes a burning mouth sensation.
♦ Allergies to dental filling materials such as composite or mercury, or oral galvanism (dissimilar metals placed in the mouth).
♦ Dry mouth due to Sjorgren's syndrome, a condition that causes dryness of the eyes and mouth.
♦ Nutritional deficiencies such as iron, zinc, folate and vitamins B_1, B_2, B_6, B_9, B_{12} and niacin.
♦ Candidiasis (yeast infection).
♦ Allergies to toothpaste (sodium lauryl sulfate, other chemicals or flavorings).
♦ Allergies to mouthwash (alcohol, chemicals or flavorings).
♦ Food allergies.

- Conditions such as gastric reflux, pernicious anemia, diabetes, rheumatoid arthritis, hypothyroidism, or thyroid disease.
- Problem in the nerves that control taste and pain in the tongue.
- Reaction to medications.
- Psychological dysfunction, which may not be a cause but a by-product of the pain and other symptoms associated with burning mouth syndrome.
- Chronic pain conditions such as myofascial pain or TMJ.
- Hormonal changes, usually due to menopause.
- Nighttime teeth grinding.
- Damage to the taste areas of the central nervous system, possibly due to trauma or viral infections.

Although nutritional deficiencies and high glucose levels are commonly present with burning mouth syndrome, studies have not thus far supported these factors as actual causes.

Treatment of Burning Mouth Syndrome

To receive the appropriate treatment, it is very important to single out the cause of burning mouth syndrome. Start with the simple causes and make an assessment list to help find the root of your symptoms. Below is a sample questionnaire that may help you to ferret out the cause.

1. When did you first notice symptoms associated with burning mouth syndrome? Note if the onset of symptoms was associated with any of the items listed below.
2. Do you wear dentures? If you do, get a dental check-up to make sure they are not irritating your mouth.
3. Did you notice symptoms after a dental visit when you had some new fillings or crowns placed in your mouth? If so, ask

your dentist if you have dissimilar metals in your mouth, and consider changing them to one type of material.

4. Could your toothpaste or mouthwash be at fault? Discontinue any toothpaste that contains sodium lauryl sulfate. This is a very strong industrial cleanser and many people are allergic to it. On the other hand, if your toothpaste contains sodium laurel sarcocinate, you should be safe. This is a mild cleanser used for contact lens cleansers and baby shampoos and is not associated with allergies. Discontinue any mouthwash with alcohol.

5. Do you wake up in the morning with soreness in your jaw area? If so, you may be clenching or grinding your teeth. Ask your dentist for a **night guard**.

6. Are medications the cause? (See the box below.)

7. Could alcohol be the source of the problem? If you do drink, discontinue using alcohol for several weeks to determine if that eases your symptoms.

Common causes of burning mouth

The following list of medications may cause burning mouth or dry mouth . If you are taking any of these and you noticed the onset of your symptoms after you began taking them, ask your doctor to consider a substitute medication. See also Chapter Five for a list, by medical condition, of medications that can cause dry mouth.

- Amitriptyline hydrochloride (Elavil, Endep)
- Doxepin (Adapin, Sinequan)
- Nortriptyline (Aventyl, Pamelor)
- Paroxetine (Paxil)
- Sertraline (Zoloft)
- Cyclobenzaprine (Cycloflex, Flexeril)

- Maprotiline (Ludiomil)
- Trazodone (Desyrel, Trazon, Trialodine)
- Fluoxetine Hydrochloride (Prozac)
- Nefazodone (Serzone)
- Tizanidine(Zanaflex)

The following prescription drugs have the strongest xerostomic (dry mouth) side effects:

- Zantac (ranitidine)
- Xanax (alprazolam)
- Seldane (terfenadine)
- Naprosyn (naproxen)
- Prozac (fluoxetine)
- Proventil (albuterol)
- Tagamet (cimetidine)
- Dyazide (triameterene)
- Hydrochlorthiazide

The following over-the-counter drugs have the greatest capability of causing dry mouth:

- Laxatives—Chronulac, Phospho-Soda
- Antinauseants—Dramamine
- Cold and Allergy Products
- Antihistimines
- Antidiarrheals—Loperamide

Other drugs that may cause dry mouth:

- Tobacco
- Marijuana
- Cocaine
- Heroin
- Amphetamines

I hope that these questions help you to identify the reason for your burning mouth syndrome and that removing the cause eliminates your problem. In the meantime, there are several actions that may be helpful in relieving discomfort from burning mouth syndrome:

- **Capsaicin**, extract from red chili peppers, has been shown to be helpful. See the box below for directions.
- Klonopin or Librium could be helpful and may be prescribed by your doctor to relieve burning mouth syndrome.
- Cool off your mouth by sipping on water with ice chips.
- If the cause is nutritional deficiencies, take the appropriate action to give your body the food and supplements it needs.
- If allergy is found to be the cause, determine what food(s) could be the culprits.
- If thrush (candidiasis) or other oral conditions are present, seek medical treatment.
- If you have uncontrolled diabetes, you need to consult your doctor for this and many other important reasons.

How to use capsaicin

Capsaicin is applied in topical form on the site of pain four times a day for four weeks. Another suggested way to use capsaicin is to mix two teaspoons water and one teaspoon Tabasco sauce and rinse your mouth with this for approximately fifteen seconds every two to three hours several days. It may burn initially, but some people have reported relief. Increase the strength of capsaicin to a maximum of 1:1 dilution, as tolerated.

We have yet to discover a clear, underlying cause or definitive treatment for burning mouth syndrome. One clinical research project in Italy tested sixty patients with constant burning mouth syndrome in a controlled double blind study for two months. They compared alpha-lipoic acid with a placebo form of treatment. They concluded that following the alpha-lipoic acid treatment, the symptoms had improved and were maintained during the one-year follow-up. Alpha-lipoic acid is an antioxidant that is said to target mitochondria of cells to get rid of harmful free radicals. The best advice I can offer is to encourage you to attempt to find the cause in your situation and to experiment with a variety of treatment options to find what works best for you.

10

COLD SORES

Take Time for Relief

Cold sores, also called **fever blisters**, come without any warning. You feel a hard spot that tingles and itches, and in a day or two a fluid-filled blister appears. Cold sores usually occur on the edges of your lip or nose, but they can appear almost anywhere on the face. This is one way to distinguish these sores from **canker sores**, which more than likely only appear inside the mouth. Cold sores are different from canker sores, which are discussed in Chapter Six. Cold sores are very annoying, painful sores which won't go away quickly and usually appear at the most inopportune time.

As we'll soon discuss, cold sores appear to be related in many instances with an impaired immune system, which also seems to lie at the root of fibromyalgia and many of the problems it causes. Not everyone with cold sores has fibromyalgia, or visa versa, but it's not unlikely that fibromyalgia predisposes a person to the occurrence of cold sores. Moreover, if you do develop cold sores, they can probably be aggravated by your fibromyalgia, so it's all the more important that you treat their symptoms as effectively as possible.

It's very important to know that the **herpes simplex virus** causes cold sores and that they are contagious. Kissing and sharing food utensils are two methods of transmitting cold sores to others. Even sharing towels or linen with an infected person can pass along the virus. The blisters are filled with virus and frequent hand washing is recommended every time the cold sores are touched.

The initial infection is usually acquired by direct contact with someone who has the infected blisters (primary herpetic **stomatitis**). The initial outbreak may be accompanied with flu-like symptoms such as fever, headache, and irritability. When a person is first infected, there may not be any outbreaks at that time. Statistics indicates that infected individuals experience four to five outbreaks per year. For the virus to be transmitted to someone else, it usually has to be in the active state.

Cold sores don't present a serious problem unless the infection is spread to the eye (caused by touching the sore and then the eye). This can cause ulceration of the cornea. However, individuals with an immune deficiency disorder do have to practice extra caution, because the herpes virus can spread to the brain and other parts of the central nervous system, resulting in meningitis and encephalitis.

There are two types of herpes simplex infection: herpes simplex virus one (HSV-1) and herpes simplex virus two (HSV-2). The terms "oral herpes" versus "genital herpes" distinguish where the infection appears rather than the type of virus that causes it.

Approximately sixty percent of HSV-1 sores usually appear in or around the mouth (oral herpes), while forty percent of HSV-1 infect the genitals (genital herpes), thighs, and buttocks. On the other hand, sixty percent of HSV-2 occurrences affect the genitals, thighs and buttocks, and are caused by sexual contact, while forty percent of sores in those areas are infected with HSV-1.

Estimates suggest that eighty percent of the population is infected with the herpes simplex virus, but only one-third will experience its recurrent effects. For the remainder, the virus particles remain asleep in their nerve tissues. In the lips and face, they "sleep" in the trigeminal nerve ganglia (the nerve that services the face). Once reactivated, they travel from the nerve to the site where they develop. The area where the sore appears is a location that is serviced by the same nerve, giving the virus easy access to the area.

Although we don't know exactly what triggers the onset of sores, research studies have identified some possible factors, including:

+ Physical stress
+ Fatigue
+ Emotional stress
+ Compromised immune system
+ Menstruation, pregnancy, or menopause
+ Cold, flu, or other illness
+ Excessive exposure to the sun

In addition, some studies suggest foods high in **arginine** and low in **lysine** tend to increase outbreaks of blisters. Such foods include chocolate, peanuts, peas, nuts, seeds, or caffeine.

Whatever its cause, once the initial hard spot is felt, a blister appears within twelve to twenty-four hours. Within forty-eight to seventy-two hours, the blister enlarges and ruptures. As the blister dries up, a yellow crust forms. The crust or scab falls off, and the redness slowly goes away. The duration of its course, if there are no complications, is three weeks or less.

Once you have the virus in your body, it remains dormant after the outbreak. There is no consensus on what causes sores to reappear. The virus may reactivate because of some change in your immune system or some particularly stressful situation. In some cases the virus never reappears. In others, sores reoccur periodically and are referred to as "recurrent herpes simplex infections."

Easing Cold Sore Symptoms

There is no treatment for cold sores, and they generally clear up within fourteen to twenty-one days. In the meantime, to help with the symptoms you may want to follow the following steps:

◆ Let the problem take its course. Do not pull the scab off, scratch, pick, or squeeze the blister.

◆ During initial stages, apply ice on the cold sore for three to five minutes every hour. It's suggested that this will lower the metabolic rate, and resist the development of the sore. Ice can also decrease pain, itching, and burning.

◆ Apply hot or cold compresses to blisters for pain relief.

◆ Tannic acid, found in tea, is thought to possess antiviral properties. Placing a tea bag on cold sores at the onset of symptoms may minimize development. To try this therapy, place a moistened tea bag on the sore for a few minutes every hour.

◆ Aloe vera rubbed on a blister will help hasten healing.

◆ I don't normally recommend alcohol-based mouthwashes, but a cotton swab saturated with an alcohol-based mouthwash and dabbed on the blister two to three times a day will usually dry it up within three days.

◆ A cotton swab dabbed in hydrogen peroxide or alcohol and applied daily to the area will help dry the blisters more quickly.

◆ During outbreaks on the lips, lip balms will help prevent cracking and bleeding of sores. Lip balms may contain petrolatum allantoin or lanolin.

◆ Once a crust forms, apply vitamin E oil with a cotton swab to enhance healing.

◆ A number of clinical studies have found that lysine may help prevent and decrease outbreaks of herpes simplex infections. The dosage range for possible prevention of herpes simplex virus recurrence is 500 mg to three grams daily, with the average dose being 1,000 mg daily.

- Over-the-counter pain medications such as acetaminophen may help with pain during the outbreak of sores.
- Over-the-counter creams and ointments can provide comfort, but not healing. Most only help relieve the symptoms of pain, itching, and burning. The active ingredients in products that limit cold sore symptoms via a numbing agent may include: tetracaine, benzocaine, lidocaine, benzyl alcohol, camphor, and phenol.
- Some over-the-counter medications inhibit growth of the virus and therefore may help limit the severity and the length of the outbreak. Most of these contain the drug docosanol.
- Another category of over-the-counter drugs aims to promote healing with anti-viral ingredients. These products may contain zinc, lysine, phenol, and tannic acid. Some contain anti-bacterial agents, which will not affect healing, but may prevent a secondary bacterial infection.
- A drug called acyclovir (Zovirax) is said to be effective in treating herpes simplex. The oral form is more effective than cream.
- Penciclovir (Denavir), a prescription drug, is the first cold sore medication approved by the FDA. Its manufacturer says that it lessens the pain and speeds up healing of cold sores. Other prescription anti-viral medications that are sometimes prescribed to control outbreaks include valcyclovir (Valtrex), Viroxyn, and famciclovir (Famivir).

What You Can Do to Prevent Cold Sore Outbreaks

The following steps are suggestions to help prevent and minimize recurrent outbreaks, and passing the virus to others:

- Avoid contact such as kissing or touching blisters of people with active cold sores.

- Do not share any items such as food, silverware, towels, or linen.
- Wash your hands before touching anyone if you have a blister present.
- Sunscreen in the form of SPF 15 or greater, or zinc oxide will help prevent outbreaks. Injury to the lips may be one way to trigger outbreaks. Moisturizing lip balm will help reduce chapping, and therefore cracking lips.
- Eating a well balanced diet of vegetables and protein has been shown to be helpful.
- Diets high in lysine and low in arginine ratios can be helpful in preventing outbreaks of herpes simplex. These include:
  - Dairy products such as plain low fat yogurt
  - Mango, apples, and apricots
  - Margarine
  - Fish, red meat
  - Brewer's yeast
  - Beans, peas, and lentils

11

CANKER SORES

Coping Strategies

Have patience with all things, but chiefly have patience
with yourself. Do not lose courage in considering your own
imperfections but instantly set about remedying them—
every day begins the task anew.
—*Saint Francis de Sales*

Canker sores are painful, annoying, and can make eating very
unpleasant. These sores are a type of mouth ulcers called
"recurrent **aphthous ulcers**." The term aphtha means "ulcer." For
many years the term has been used to describe ulcers that are
painful and tend to recur. They appear on the tongue, soft palate,
inside the cheeks or lips, and at the base of the gums. The sores are
typically appear whitish with a red edge or halo. While cold sores,
discussed in Chapter Five, are very contagious, canker sores are
not. Another difference between the two is that canker sores show
up inside the mouth, while cold sores (herpes simplex) most often
appear around the lips, nose, or genitals.

As with cold sores, the immune system basis of canker sores
should be of particular interest to if you have fibromyalgia. The link
is hazy because science still faces many unanswered questions
both about fibromyalgia and other immune system-related disorders including canker sores. In general, though, canker sores can
present a special problem for you if you have fibromyalgia.

At least ten percent of the population suffers from canker sores. Women are more susceptible than men, and their incidence seems to run in families; children of parents who have canker sores have a ninety percent chance of developing them. Once they appear, canker sores will continue to return due to certain triggers. As with cold sores, the precise mechanism that causes canker sores is unclear. They apparently result from an immune system response in which the appearance of an unidentified or potentially hazardous molecule activates a concentration of lymphocytes (a type of white blood cell) in the affected area. The lymphocytes' attack forms a canker sore. We don't yet understand why the immune system behaves in this way in some people and not in others.

Canker sores can be triggered by any of the following:

◆ Irritants in the mouth, such as certain toothpaste ingredients. Research suggests that sodium lauryl sulfate (SLS), used as a foaming agent in most toothpastes and mouthwashes, can trigger formation of canker sores.
◆ Mechanical trauma can also activate the appearance of these ulcers. The trauma could be from a bite on a cheek or tongue, or an irritating temporary crown, filling, or ill-fitting dentures. Chewing a hard French bread or pizza crust could also traumatize the mouth and cause a canker sore to flare up.
◆ Emotional stress affects our health in many ways including canker sore outbreaks.
◆ Compromised immune system can allow canker sores to develop.
◆ Certain nutritional deficiencies have also been found to contribute to the onset of canker sores. These deficiencies might include:
  ✧ Vitamin B_1, B_2, B_6, B_{12}, and C
  ✧ Zinc, folic acid, iron, selenium, calcium
◆ Breakouts could also be brought about by allergies. Some of the most common types of substances responsible for breakouts are:

- ✧ Dairy products such as cheeses or milk
- ✧ Lemons, oranges, pineapples, tomatoes, or strawberries
- ✧ Chocolate, shellfish, soy, vinegar
- ✧ Cinnamonaldehyde (a flavoring agent)
- ✧ Benzoic acid (a preservative)
- ✧ Metals used for dental caps, crowns, or fillings, such as nickel, copper, or tin.
- ◆ Hormonal changes during menstruation or menopause may trigger cold sores or cause their remission.
- ◆ Certain medical conditions are related and associated to canker sores, including:
  - ✧ Behcet's disease
  - ✧ Crohn's disease
  - ✧ Ulcerative colitis (five to twenty percent of those with canker sore outbreaks have been linked to this disease).
  - ✧ Malabsorption syndromes such as gluten-sensitive enteropathy, and inflammatory bowel diseases
- ◆ Medications that may cause the sores to appear include non-steroidal anti-inflammatory drugs (**NSAID**s), beta-blockers, and chemotherapeutic agents.

Treatment Options

There is no cure for canker sores, and the sores usually heal within twenty-one days if left to resolve on their own. However, there are several different ways to treat the symptoms, which can include the painful sores themselves and the tingling or burning sensation prior to their appearance. Fever, fatigue, or swollen glands may also be present, but may not always be related to canker sores. You should contact your physician if the sores last longer than three weeks, if you have high fever with the canker sores, or you have difficulty drinking fluids.

Over-the-Counter Medications

- ◆ Over-the-counter products act as bandages that help to protect the ulcer from further irritation. Two of these products are Orabase and Zilactin.
- ◆ To help cleanse the ulcerations, rinse with astringents such as hydrogen peroxide. Mix equal parts of two percent hydrogen peroxide with warm water and rinse at least three to four times a day. Rinsing with denatured alcohol in mouthwashes such as Listerine (non-mint for those on guai protocol) is also helpful. Do not use alcohol mouthwash as a routine rinse, only with the outbreak of these sores. If you don't see any improvement within two to three days, discontinue.
- ◆ To help with the pain canker sores can cause, topical anesthetics such as two percent Viscous Xylocaine; Benadryl, Kaopectate 50:50 suspension, and silver nitrate are helpful. Kaopecate with Benadryl, and Orabase with Benzocaine act as covering on the sores and will temporarily numb them, relieving pain.
- ◆ A half and half mixture of magnesia and benadryl allergy liquid swished in the mouth three to four times a day is also helpful for pain relief.
- ◆ Rinsing with saline solution can be helpful.
- ◆ Over-the-counter pain medications such as acetaminophen.
- ◆ Herbs and supplements should be taken with the advice of a physician trained in these fields, but several herbal and supplement products appear to provide some relief.
  - ✧ L-Lysine is believed to help prevent outbreaks and hasten healing of sores. The suggested dose is 500 mg once or twice a day (depending on how often outbreaks occur).
  - ✧ Vitamin B complex, in combination with vitamin C, enhances healing.
  - ✧ Tea tree oil may be useful as an antiseptic.

Prescription drugs for canker sores

The following must be used under direction of your physician or dentist:

◆ Prescription antibacterial mouthwashes containing chlorhexidine gluconate will speed up healing. These come in several brand names such as Oris and Peridex. Most contain salicylates. For salicylate-free chlorhexidine gluconate mouthrinse, contact Mulberry Pharmacy in Florida (877) 425-1101. However, your dentist must fax them a prescription in order for them to send you the salicylate-free form of this mouth rinse. There are no side effects with this rinse, except that with prolonged use some staining of the teeth may occur.

◆ Tetracycline is a systemic and topical antibiotic. Dissolving the contents of a 250 mg tetracycline capsule in thirty milliliters (six teaspoons) of water and swishing and swallowing it six times a day may be helpful. An alternative is to swish and swallow tetracycline syrup, 125 milligrams per teaspoon, four times a day. With fibromyalgia, all forms of antibiotics should be taken with caution. Long-term use may lead to yeast infection.

◆ Levamisole has also been recommended. However, it may have side effects of neutropenia (abnormally low number of neutrophils, a form of white blood cells). Thalidomide (not available in the United States) has also been shown to be beneficial.

◆ Apthasol (amlexanox) is marketed specifically for the treatment of canker sores. It has anti-allergic and anti-inflammatory properties. However, regular use has not shown to reduce recurrence of the ulcers. Apthasol comes in a paste and forms a film over the sore to protect the surface and allow the active ingredient to be in direct contact with the sore.

The manufacturer recommends applying it four times a day, after each meal and before bedtime, until healing occurs. The manufacturer warns not to use this drug if you have immune system problems.

◆ Kenalog (triamcinolone acetonide) is a synthetic corticosteroid, which has anti-inflammatory properties. The purpose of kenalog is to keep the canker sore from advancing. It is added to a paste called Orabase, and then placed on the ulcer. The manufacturer warns that you should take this with caution if you have high blood pressure, osteoporosis, or kidney problems.

◆ Other anti-inflammatory prescription drugs in the form of corticosteriods include Fluocinonice (Lidex), betamethasone (Diprolene), and clobetasol (Temovate). When using any corticosteroids, make sure you don't cover the cold sore with a bandage. Covering it increases the amount of drug the body absorbs.

Preventing Canker Sore Outbreaks

◆ Avoid spicy, acidic, salty, and abrasive foods during outbreaks. Other types of foods to avoid are hard crusty breads and pizzas and potato chips. Avoid acidic drinks such as tomato juice, citrus juices, and alcoholic drinks. When sores are present, eat soft foods.

◆ Eat hard, crusty foods very carefully to avoid trauma which may trigger canker sores. Apply ice to the sores for pain relief.

◆ Avoid toothpaste that contains sodium lauryl sulfate. Some toothpaste contains sodium lauryth succinate as a mild cleanser. This ingredient is safe and I recommend using toothpastes that contain it.

◆ Reduce stress or learn how to manage it better.

- See your dentist and treat any broken, sharp and old crowns or fillings. Have any ill-fitting dentures adjusted so they are comfortable and don't rub against your tongue, cheeks, or gums.
- Practice good oral hygiene habits daily. Food left between the teeth and gums may eventually trigger a sore. Also, use a soft toothbrush, and clean your mouth gently to avoid irritation and trauma.

12

MERCURY FILLINGS

What You Should Believe

Three things cannot long be hidden,
the sun, the moon, and the truth.
—*Confucious*

"**Could my silver/mercury** fillings be contributing to or even causing my fibromyalgia?" This is a question I am asked very frequently. Due to extensive media exposure, the mercury filling controversy—safe or unsafe—has climbed to a fever-pitch in the last twenty years. There have been numerous television news programs, such as CBS's *60 Minutes*, "exposing" toxins in our mouths that could be poisoning us. It's no wonder Americans want to know if these reports are fact or quackery; millions of people have mercury-containing amalgam fillings in their mouths and millions more will be getting these types of fillings from their dentists.

As you'll read in this chapter, my professional opinion—based on considerable thought and research—is that amalgam fillings pose no discernable risk, but that there are valid reasons for patients to opt for alternative filling materials.

What your dentist refers to as "**amalgam**" is a mixture of approximately forty to sixty percent mercury, and the rest a combination of copper, tin, and silver. Smaller amounts of zinc, palladium, or indium may also be present in the mixture. Amalgam is mixed before placing it in the mouth as a filling in a tooth. The mixture consists of "elemental" mercury and a combination of the metals listed. The American Dental Association maintains that although elemental or "organic" mercury is toxic, once it is mixed with the other metals it becomes chemically bound to the other metals, making it safe.

I once heard a very interesting comparison that's useful in understanding amalgam risk. Elemental hydrogen is an explosive gas. Elemental oxygen is a gas that supports combustion. When combined, however, they form water, which has neither of these characteristics. Saying that amalgam will poison you is like saying that drinking water will make you explode and burst into flames. Some people remain unconvinced, however.

Holistic dentists, for example, maintain that the friction produced by chewing releases molecules from the amalgam filling in the form of elemental mercury, which then enter the body. They also argue that mercury vapor is generated from the amalgam filling.

The history of amalgam goes back some 150 years when it was developed by a chemist as a filling material option for people who could not afford gold. From the start, there was controversy in the dental profession about amalgam fillings. However, most of the alarm and concern began in 1989 when the Environmental Protection Agency declared mercury amalgam to be a toxic substance. Reporter Morley Safer broadcast the EPA report on *60 Minutes* featuring interviews with dentist Dr. Hal Huggins, who has a clinic in Colorado Springs, Colorado.

The Amalgam Controversy Heats Up

When this controversy first began in the 1980s, I became very interested in knowing the truth about what I was placing in my patients' mouths. I attended numerous seminars (including courses from Hal Huggins) and carefully studied the pros and cons of the issue. I removed mercury fillings from patients who had multiple sclerosis, Parkinson's disease, cancer, and other serious diseases, who had been referred to me by holistic physicians. For the next ten years I followed all of Hal Huggins's methods, looking for a "dental connection" between disease and health. This chapter will present to you all the facts from both sides and my conclusions regarding the mercury controversy

Dr. Huggins published a book titled *It's All In Your Head* in 1985. In his book, he indicates that his interest in amalgam began when Olympio Pinto, CD, from Rio de Janeiro, told him that removing silver/mercury fillings cured many diseases such as leukemia, Hodgkin's disease, and bowel disorders. In his book, he states "I started to observe what happened to patients' body chemistries when these mercury-laden fillings were removed." However, he does not indicate how he "observed" what the results of his patients' body chemistries were. This lack of detail made me curious about the research methods he had used to arrive at his conclusions.

The Dubious Findings of Holistic Dentistry

According to Huggins, just about every disease known to science has a connection to mercury fillings. He writes that mercury can interfere with nerve impulse transmission, causing organs to get wrong messages. He concludes that this may be related to frequent memory problems, contribute to numbness and tingling of the extremities, and that mercury can become attached to hormones and deactivate them.

He also asserts that chronic fatigue syndrome and fibromyalgia have a mercury connection. He reasons that when mercury binds to the oxygen-carrying part of hemoglobin in the blood, the hemoglobin level may look normal, but its ability to transport oxygen is hampered by mercury sitting on the transportation area.

Following Huggins, holistic dentistry became a subculture within the dental community. Other dentists such as Michael

Ziff, DDS, David Eggleston, DDS, and David Kennedy, DDS, became very vocal about mercury and other issues such as root canals.

To find toxic levels of mercury in the body, holistic dentists recommend that certain tests should be performed and that fillings must be removed according to a particular protocol. The Dental Filling Compatibility or Blood Compatibility Testing is intended to measure serum compatibility. With this test, a sample of blood is drawn and specially prepared. It's mixed with nearly a hundred dental chemicals that are included in over 1,000 dental products to produce a test result:

1. High reactivity—don't use.
2. Moderate reactivity—use only if you have to.
3. Least reactivity—most compatible with your body.

However, according to Robert S. Baratz, MD, DDS, PhD, in an article titled "Serum Compatibility Testing," nothing in the test actually shows any form of "compatibility" of the tested substances with the person's serum. Nor does the test have anything to do with immunity or the immune system. The "positive" reactions are nonspecific chemical reactions that have no practical significance.

Other Tests for Mercury Poisoning:

◆ Urine testing—This is a fairly reliable indicator of heavy metal exposure. However, this test is usually ordered by holistic dentists or physicians on a urine sample obtained after the patient takes a chelation drug (a chemical compound that combines with mercury and other heavy metals) called DMSA or DMPS. Everyone has some mercury in the body, but when DMSA or DMPS are taken, they can produce an abnormally high reading, because the chelation agent binds with small amounts of mercury throughout the body and forces them to be excreted.

♦ Hair Analysis—A commercial hair analysis laboratory can generate a computerized report by analyzing a sample of hair (the nape of the neck is the recommended source). The report indicates in micrograms the amount of mercury found in the body.

Unfortunately, there are no universally accepted standards by which to evaluate mercury levels in hair samples, because hair thickness, density, shape, and growth rate vary so much. The determination of harmful amounts is usually based on a single laboratory's estimation of average vs. harmful samples that it has tested. Because mercury can enter the body from water, air, and many foods and products (see end of this chapter), even if hair analysis were standardized, it would be difficult to determine the source of the mercury.

♦ Stool Testing—This test may indicate that mercury was present in the gastrointestinal tract, but it cannot measure and analyze the source of exposure.

Some Very Strange Machines

To further complicate matters, Huggins indicates that as he began to remove the fillings from his patients, he learned that some fillings have varying degrees of "negative electrical current" and must be removed in a proper sequence or their removal may cause more harm. The fillings have to be taken out within thirty days and all schedules have to be made in accordance with a seven/ fourteen/ twenty-one day immune cycle; otherwise, Huggins warned, "You might create an autoimmune disease, you otherwise have never had." His protocol indicates that patients must be scheduled "to have appointments of two hours on Monday, Wednesday, and Friday on one week, and Tuesday, Thursday, and Saturday the next week. If all the 'removal' procedures are performed within thirty days, chances are a bit better than if sixty days are required, and if you are having one filling a month replaced for financial reasons, forget it. You will probably feel no improvement. Save up for a year, and then have it all done within thirty days."

I see absolutely no scientific or other reason why such a schedule would make any difference, except for the obvious fact that if you had appointments every day, you would get very tired and stressed. I have never seen one of my patients who did not have all their treatment completed within Dr. Huggins's prescribed thirty-day cycle who developed any autoimmune disease.

Looking further into this protocol, I purchased an "Amalgemeter" from Dr. Huggins and proceeded to measure the currents from the amalgam fillings of all my patients over a period of two years. The measurement is achieved by placing a probe on an amalgam filling while the patient holds a brass cylinder. The amperage from the probe appears on the machine. What I learned was that this process registered a flow of current due to the creation of a low-voltage circuit, nothing more. I also found that the machine was very unpredictable, with readings on the same patient, during the same appointment, differing greatly when taken only a few minutes apart. I concluded that I was unable to follow any protocol for removing fillings for the dental quadrant containing the highest negative current levels when the readings were constantly changing.

I also experimented with other types of machines recommended by holistic dentists, such as, the EAV (Electro-acupuncture according to Voll). Reinhold Voll was a German physician who combined acupuncture with "galvanic skin differentials." With the EAV, a probe was placed on certain acupuncture points on the hands. Readings from the device supposedly identified disease in remote parts of the body and a chart indicated the tooth causing the disease in the corresponding organ.

More elaborate machines, such as the Acupath 1000 and Biotron are also used by holistic physicians and naturopaths to diagnose and treat patients with **homeopathy**. Readings from these devices usually seem to result in a prescription to remove not only mercury fillings but also to extract all teeth with root canals. (Root canals are the subject of Chapter Seventeen.)

How Much Is Too Much?

The federally determined legal limit of safe mercury exposure for industrial workers is fifty micrograms per cubic meter of air for eight hours per day and fifty weeks per year. Exposure at this level will produce urine mercury levels of about 135 micrograms per liter. These levels are much higher than those in the general public but produce no symptoms and are considered safe. Most people without fillings have a maximum of five to ten micrograms per liter of mercury in their urine. Most practicing dentists have levels below ten micrograms per liter, even though they are exposed to mercury vapor when placing or removing amalgam fillings and typically have amalgams in their own teeth. Thus, even with their ongoing exposure, the maximum levels found in dentists are only twice those of their patients—and most dentists have the same levels as most patients. These are far below the levels known to affect health, even in a minor way.

Fillings are, of course, not the only source of mercury exposure. Mercury is a fairly common element in the earth's crust and occurs naturally in water, food, and air. Even without amalgam fillings, everyone has small but measurable blood and urine levels of mercury. Amalgam fillings raise these levels slightly, but this has no clinical significance. Studies indicate that fish consumption is a major source of methyl mercury exposure. Fish pick up mercury as they feed in streams and oceans. Micro-organisms in the ocean transform mercury into the toxic elemental form of methyl mercury. This "organic" form is absorbed by the fish as they feed on the micro-organisms. Most of this mercury falls into the ocean from coal-powered factories. Larger fish and those that eat other fish contain more mercury. Fish highest in mercury include: sharks, rays, swordfish, tilefish, and king mackerel. The FDA recommends that children, pregnant and breastfeeding women should not eat more than twelve ounces of these types of fish per week. Seafood with lower amounts of mercury include: shellfish, trout, catfish, blue crab, lobster, prawns, and salmon. Some environmental groups list most fish as mercury-contaminated and recommend that seafood consumption be limited to once per week.

Separating Myths from Facts

This chapter began by asking, "Could my silver/mercury fillings be contributing to or even causing my fibromyalgia?" Let's summarize what we now know:

1. Myth: Fillings wear out and disappear over time, which means they are vaporizing or being deposited in my organs.

   Fact: In reality, amalgam fillings usually do not wear out, but either corrode, **pit**, or fracture. Many people had their amalgam fillings placed when they were children and they are often still in place far into their adult years. If a filling breaks and is swallowed whole, it will be excreted.

2. Myth: Mercury affects my immune system and weakens it. It also blocks DBH (dopamine-beta-hydroxylase), which is a catalyst in the body that helps make noradrenalin (NA) **neurotransmitter**. Low levels of neurotransmitters cause fatigue and depression. Therefore, mercury in dental fillings causes chronic fatigue and fibromyalgia due to the effect it has on this neurotransmitter through the catalyst DBH.

Fact: It has been found that some people with fibromyalgia have alterations in some neurotransmitters, including serotonin, estrogen, and thyroid hormones. **Serotonin** is especially important, and is often linked with depression, migraines, and gastrointestinal distress. Another neurotransmitter that is sometimes found in abnormal levels in some people with fibromyalgia is "substance P." This chemical is found in people suffering from pain, stress, anxiety, and depression. Whether the abnormal hormone levels are the result of the effects of pain and stress on the central nervous system or the cause of fibromyalgia is yet not fully understood.

Fibromyalgia resembles **autoimmune disorder**s such as rheumatoid arthritis and systemic lupus erythematosus. The cause of these diseases is a faulty immune system that produces factors that attack proteins in the body's own tissue. Similar factors (**autoantibodies**) which affect neurological and hormonal systems have been found in many fibromyalgia patients. However, there is no evidence that a faulty immune system is a primary cause of fibromyalgia. In fact, we still don't know what exactly causes fibromyalgia.

3. Myth: Mercury can disrupt the sleep cycle. Mercury and other heavy metals affect certain hormones (noradrenalin) which interrupt the sleep cycle.

   Fact: Some researchers have suggested that disturbed sleep patterns, rather than being a symptom of fibromyalgia, could be a possible cause. Low levels of a particular hormone called somatomedin C are usually found in the blood of individuals with fibromyalgia. This hormone is secreted during Stage Four sleep (the deepest sleep phase) and is essential for the body to rebuild itself. No studies have linked the levels of this hormone to mercury.

Alternatives to Mercury Fillings

No major organization that focuses its research on specific chronic conditions such as cancer, Parkinson's, and fibromyalgia has established any relationship between those diseases and mercury amalgam fillings. Any hint of a connection would be immediately published and exhaustively researched. So far, though, the only claims come from holistic dentists who insist that the most threatening and dangerous source of mercury toxicity is the amalgam filling.

So, why would someone want to change their mercury amalgam fillings, and if they did, what are their options? One good reason is to want a more beautiful smile. Not long ago, most dentists resisted the change to white resin-type filling materials because they felt they could not compare to amalgam for strength and durability. However, over the years dental science has become more technologically sophisticated and the filling material choices have improved significantly.

Cosmetic concerns and demands have been one of the reasons that more choices and improvement in dental materials have appeared. Given the choice, patients prefer fillings that match the color of natural teeth rather than the grayish black appearance of amalgam. Many patients now specifically request the non-mercury fillings and will, if necessary, even change dentists to get them.

Although the demand for the non-mercury fillings is increasing, dental insurance companies have not caught up with all the demand for them. Most of the plans only cover amalgam fillings and patients have to pay the difference if they want the white fillings, which are generally more expensive. However, as research continues to support the effectiveness of white resin fillings and manufacturers improve their durability, the insurance plans will surely take notice—a few, in fact, currently cover their cost.

For the present, dentists and their patients are weighing all their options. Amalgam fillings have been around for more than 150 years. Amalgam is durable, inexpensive, and covered by all

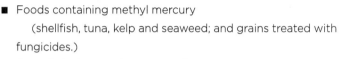

Sources of Mercury Exposure

Mercury exposure has many sources. Consider all the sources from which you could get mercury exposure and think twice before spending thousands of dollars removing your amalgam fillings. Sources of mercury include:

- Foods containing methyl mercury
  (shellfish, tuna, kelp and seaweed; and grains treated with fungicides.)
- Some hair dyes, and waterproof mascaras
- Medications, including over-the-counter antiseptics and first-aid preparations
- Psoriasis preparations
- Fungicides
- Acne preparations
- Bleaching creams
- Eye preparations
- Nasal drops and sprays
- Throat lozenges
- Hemorrhoid ointments and suppositories
- Vaginal jellies, tablets, and douches
- Hair tonic (mercuric chloride)
- Veterinary preparations
- Household chemicals, such as paints, tile cements, lead mercury solder
- Garden seed fungicides, protectants, and disinfectants

insurance plans. **Composite** resin fillings are also durable, resistant to fracture, and have excellent aesthetic appeal. The disadvantage is that they may shrink slightly over time, thereby permitting decay.

Gold is another long-standing choice for a filling material. Gold is very durable and leak-resistant, and allergies to it are rare. It is expensive, however, is unattractive, and conducts heat and cold. Porcelain filling materials have excellent aesthetics, moderate durability, and no known allergic reactions. However, they are just as expensive as the gold fillings.

As a patient, it's wise to remain well informed on the options and then choose the filling material that is suitable for you. You now have a range of choices, not just gray, black or "silver" fillings. However, don't get pressured into thinking that you must remove all of your amalgam fillings and pay thousands of dollars for testing to determine what materials should be used.

I stopped using amalgam fillings in my office many years ago. The reason was that the white fillings looked nicer and were just as durable. I recommend that my patients replace their old amalgams, when they need to be replaced, with a more cosmetic type of white filling or gold.

13

ORAL HYGIENE BASICS

Brushing, Flossing, and Beyond

Archaeologists have found dental cleaning tools going back to the Stone Age, when small sticks or twigs mashed at one end were used to clean teeth. This proves that even many centuries ago our ancestors knew the importance of oral hygiene. We've become more sophisticated now and know the reasons why proper oral hygiene is so important. Periodontal (gum) disease not only attacks the bone and gums and leads to tooth loss, but can also increase the risk of heart disease and stroke. It can also lead to infection. a significant risk in people with immune systems compromised by fibromyalgia. Bacteria are the enemies that attack and destroy the supporting structures of our teeth. The only way to fight these enemies is to know how they function and what actions and tools we need to fight back.

Plaque

Plaque—bacteria living in a thin film on the surface of teeth and oral tissues are the main cause of periodontal (gum) disease and tooth decay. Prevention is the simplest way to stop the beginning stages of gum disease (gingivitis) and tooth decay from advancing to root canals and tooth loss. One important aspect of prevention is proper home oral hygiene. To start, you will need certain tools for proper oral hygiene:

◆ Soft toothbrush (manual or power)
◆ Toothpaste
◆ Floss
◆ Tongue cleaner
◆ Mouthwash or mouth rinse
◆ Toothbrush sterilizer

The home hygiene regimen is simple: floss first to remove the debris from between the teeth and under the gums. Follow by brushing and lastly, clean your tongue.

Toothbrushes

The first bristle toothbrush came from China. Europe adopted bristle brushes for teeth cleaning in the seventeenth century. The first electric toothbrush was introduced in the late 1800s, but wasn't developed fully until just after World War II. However, these devices weren't available in the United States until the 1960s.

Today, there are many varieties of toothbrushes available in various sizes, shapes, manual- and power-operated types. Both manual and power brushes are effective. Power-operated toothbrushes used to be very expensive, but today they are almost as inexpensive as manual toothbrushes. It's a matter of personal preference which kind will motivate you to clean better. A brand-new electric toothbrush that's very high tech with lots of gadgets such as Sonicare may get you all excited and make your teeth and gums squeaky-clean. The question is: Will you be as motivated once the novelty wears off?

One very positive aspect of power toothbrushes is that you don't have to worry if you're brushing right or wrong. All you have to do is hold the handle and move it from tooth to tooth, and it will clean the teeth. For this reason alone, studies show a reduction in plaque following a shift from manual brushing to power brushing. Of course, if you rush and don't hold the brush on each tooth for at least one full second, then it won't get the benefit you should from the brushing. Power brushes are also very useful for people who place too much pressure on their teeth and brush too hard when using a manual toothbrush. Power toothbrushes are good for people with braces and individuals who lack manual dexterity or have any form of disability, including the elderly or those with arthritis. If you have gum disease, you may want to try a power toothbrush that's recommended by your dentist. Ultimately, though, clean teeth depend more on the brusher than the brush.

The key thing to remember about toothbrushes is that they must be soft; hard bristles may wear tooth surfaces (**abrasion**) and cause gum recession. Always brush in a forty-five degree angle at the gum line in a gentle circular motion, and clean not only the teeth, but the gums as well. Brush the teeth for a minimum of two to three minutes. Follow a consistent routine in your brushing technique. For example, begin in the upper back right side. Brush the outer surfaces as you move across to the upper back left side. From there move to the lower left side and move along to the lower right side. In other words, find a pattern that you follow when you brush and repeat it every time you brush. Brush every side of every tooth including the tongue side, palate side, and chewing surfaces of the teeth. When you are through brushing, run your tongue around your teeth. They should feel clean and smooth. If you missed any areas you will feel a film; go over those areas with your toothbrush until they feel clean.

In general, you need a brush that will reach the back teeth, with a handle that fits into your palm comfortably. Avoid a brush head that is too cumbersome. Often, a small brush head, even one that is meant for children, is suitable, especially if you have a small mouth.

Studies conducted at the University of Oklahoma School of Dentistry by Richard T. Glass, DDS, have proven that toothbrushes are breeding grounds for bacteria and can make you sick unless they are properly cleaned on a daily basis. It would, indeed, seem very unhealthy and odd to eat three meals a day with the same fork by just rinsing it under water. However, this is exactly what most people do with their toothbrushes. As if that's not bad enough, we usually store our toothbrushes in the bathroom, where every flush exposes them to airborne bacteria. You've probably heard that you should change toothbrushes every two to three months. However, when you think of the comparison with the fork, that doesn't sound too good. To adequately clean toothbrushes, there is currently only one company that manufactures the proper sterilizing instrument. The unit is called Purebrush and is only available through the Internet at www.purebrush.com or by telephone at (888) 883-4276. You can clean manual as well as power toothbrushes in this unit. The Purebrush UV-Light product is the only adequate home toothbrush purification system that kills ninety-nine and nine-tenths percent of harmful pathogens. Remember that gum disease is contagious, so don't share your toothbrush.

With electric toothbrushes, the ones with a small round brush such as Oral B are effective. However, this may be more of a personal choice and using one you like motivates you more. Remember it is the action of the bristles that clean the teeth and gums, not sonic vibrations or other claims made by some companies. Whether you use an electric or manual brush, don't apply heavy pressure to the teeth. Make sure you are thorough in cleaning the backside of the lower front teeth. The sublingual salivary gland openings are located here, and plaque tends to accumulate more heavily in this location. People tend to miss this area when brushing because it's hard to reach. You may have been told by your dentist or hygienist to clean that area better.

Flossing

Flossing is the most appropriate way to prevent decay between the teeth. Brushing alone will not prevent gum disease and tooth decay, because the bristles of a toothbrush will not reach between the teeth where bacteria hide, accumulate, and cause damage if not thoroughly removed with flossing. There are different types of floss: waxed, un-waxed, and tape. Tape is mostly used for areas where there are spaces. Your dentist will recommend which type is best for you. Floss "threaders" are used to clean under dental bridges or with braces.

Here are some tips for flossing effectively:

1. Use an arm's length (eighteen inches) of floss. Wrap it around the middle finger of one hand. Leave approximately six inches and wrap that around the middle finger of the other hand with about one inch of floss between the fingers of each hand.
2. Hold the floss firmly but not tightly so that it cuts off circulation.
3. Floss each tooth forming a "C" shape with the floss and carefully clean each side of each tooth and under the gums.
4. Introduce a new area of floss into each area.
5. Don't forget to floss behind your last molar.

Flossing removes the plaque from behind and in between your teeth that brushing misses. In general, flossing helps prevent periodontal disease by removing plaque from hard-to-reach areas.

Tongue Cleaning

Most bad breath is caused by the accumulation of bacteria on the tongue, especially the back part of the tongue. This is why cleaning the tongue is very important. You can either use your toothbrush to clean your tongue or you can buy a tongue cleaner. There are many tongue cleaners available on the market. Some are surgical steel and never have to be replaced, while others are plastic and should be replaced with the same frequency as recommended for toothbrushes.

If you use your toothbrush to clean your tongue, put slight pressure (not enough to irritate) on the brush and make strokes from the back of the tongue to the front. Make sure you have some toothpaste on the brush head.

If you are a gagger, a tongue scraper may be more useful. Before buying a tongue scraper, experiment with a small spoon. If you are successful and don't gag when cleaning your tongue with a spoon, then try one of the tongue scrapers sold at your local drug store. These come with a handle and the head is in a variety of shapes. You may want to try different ones until you find one that works best for you.

Toothpaste

The familiar collapsible tubes of toothpaste began to appear in the late 1800s and their contents consisted of soap and chalk. Many people remember their grandmothers telling them to brush with baking soda. Powdered charcoal was another popular dentifrice in the nineteenth century. One formula consisted of powdered myrrh, honey, and green sage. This was advertised not only to clean teeth, but also to fight bad breath. In 1956, Procter & Gamble developed and marketed Crest with fluoride.

Today, store shelves overflow with varieties of toothpastes that claim to solve all your dental problems. This is a multi-billion-dollar industry that seduces consumers into buying toothpaste based on what they're told in advertisements. It's important to understand what the common similarity between all of these brands is. While gels may be slightly more abrasive than pastes, most products contain the same ingredients:

Abrasives (20 percent)—to remove stains
Detergent (1–2 percent)—to cause sudsing and foaming
Binding agents (1 percent)—to add consistency
Humectants (10–30 percent)—to prevent drying

Flavoring, sweetening and coloring agents (1–5 per cent)—
taste and appearance
Preservatives (0.05–0.5 per cent)—to extend shelf life
Water

Abrasives (twenty to thirty percent). Abrasives are used as
cleaning and polishing agents. Toothpaste that is too abrasive may
wear down white fillings or make teeth too sensitive. A popular
abrasive is baking soda.

Fluoride (twenty-four percent). in toothpaste is usually in
the form of stannous fluoride, **sodium fluoride**, or monofluoride
phosphate (MFP).

Xylitol is not in all toothpastes, but it has been shown to help
prevent cavities. It also has sweetening properties.

Detergent (one to two percent). This is used for foaming, as
well as helping to loosen plaque and other debris from the tooth
surface. Examples are **sodium lauryl sulphate** and **sodium
lauryl sarcosinate**. Studies indicate sodium lauryl sulphate may
cause outbreaks of canker sores. This is an industrial detergent and
used in shampoos and many other products. Sodium lauryl sarcosinate is a mild cleanser and is preferred to the former.

For those who are on the guaifenesin protocol and must use
salicylate-free products, there are a few salicylate-free toothpastes
available, including Grace Fibro Smile Dental Products.

There are many types of toothpaste on the store shelves and
choosing one can sometimes seem overwhelming. Most adult toothpastes contain fluoride. While some are very specific in what they
accomplish, others take an all-in-one approach and claim to control
tartar, provide fluoride prevent cavities, and whiten teeth. **Pyrophosphates** are the common ingredient used as tartar control.
Some individuals may find a few of the anti-tartar ingredients to be
too strong and therefore to cause sensitivity. To determine if this is the
case, change to toothpaste that is milder and without tartar control.

Many people have receded gums and these may cause sensitivity, especially with fibromyalgia, because one of the causes for

receding gums is clenching or grinding the teeth. TMJ is common with fibromyalgia and is often aggravated by clenching and grinding the teeth. There are toothpastes with claims to help stop sensitivity in teeth. Most of these contain the ingredient potassium nitrate, which may decrease sensitivity for some people but isn't universally effective. It may take two weeks or longer before toothpaste that contains potassium nitrate begins to reduce sensitivity.

There are other treatment options for sensitive teeth due to receded gums. Daily application of fluoride gel to the area at bedtime helps decrease or stop sensitivity. Bonding the area or gum grafting are other ways to treat recession of gums. However, it is important to determine the cause first and address that; otherwise, gums will continue to recede.

A special note: hydrogen peroxide has been used by the dental profession for years to treat serious gum disease, especially one type called **acute necrotizing ulcerative gingivitis (ANUG)**, also known as "**trench mouth.**" This form of gum infection is treated with antibiotics and a thorough scaling of the teeth and roots, along with several days of hydrogen peroxide. In recent years advertisers have marketed toothpaste and mouthwashes that contain hydrogen peroxide. What the public doesn't realize is that the amount of hydrogen peroxide in many of these brands is very minimal. On the other hand, rinsing with straight hydrogen peroxide may be harmful because it can alter the bacteria in the mouth and possibly allow fungal infection (candidiasis) to flourish. Every now and then I read about homemade toothpaste recipes that combine baking soda and peroxide. Such a recipe can contribute to tooth sensitivity and sloughing of the delicate gum tissue. The baking soda, which by itself can be abrasive, can also cause the teeth to wear.

Mouthwashes and Rinses

These are designed to reduce bad breath and control bacteria, act as antiseptics, and provide a pleasant taste. When prescribed by a dentist for therapeutic purposes, they will contain agents to destroy bacteria. Some of the common active ingredients are chlorohexidine gluconate, benzoic acid, hexidine, or alcohol.

- Chlorohexidine gluconate is very effective in the treatment of gum disease, but may stain teeth with long-term use.
- Triclosan has anti-inflammatory properties.
- Cetylpyridinium chloride fights plaque through its bactericidal activity.
- Peroxide oxygenating agents destroy bacteria in plaque.
- Chlorine dioxide is supposed to reduce bad breath by reducing volatile sulfur gases.
- Phenol, thymol, tea tree oil, and eugenol are essential oils and have antibacterial properties.

When using mouthwashes or rinses, follow the instructions on the package or the recommendations of your dentist.

Water Irrigators, Toothpicks, and Other Dental Aids

Water irrigators are excellent for cleaning under and around difficult-to-clean areas. Brands such as Water Pik, Hydro Floss and others are useful for cleaning around braces, under the gums, and **implant**s.

Occasional use of toothpicks at restaurants is helpful. However, habitual toothpick use may cause wear between the teeth, increase sensitivity, and promote other problems. Toothpicks should not be made part of your oral hygiene routine. Inter-dental brushes shaped like small, fine Christmas trees are very useful for cleaning hard-to-reach areas under bridges, implants, braces, or gum pockets. They are technique-sensitive, so ask your dentist or hygienist to show you how to use them properly.

If you have **dental implant**s, it is important to take your time and make sure they are cleaned thoroughly on a daily basis. The most common problem of dental implant failure is poor oral hygiene. Dental implants come in a variety of types and are explained further in Chapter Eighteen. These are anchors placed in the jaw bone to replace lost teeth.

Chewing Gum containing sugar is not healthy for the teeth. In fact, chewing sugared gum is like bathing your teeth with acid. People with any signs of TMJ or jaw joint disorders should be warned to avoid chewing gum, or aggravated joints can become very painful. However, an occasional stick of chewing gum for fresh breath or to clean teeth between meals is refreshing.

In summary, to maintain a healthy mouth and fresh breath, practice proper home oral hygiene, see your dentist at recommended intervals, and eat a balanced diet. The following are easy to follow steps for fresh, clean breath:

At bedtime and in the morning:
1. Floss thoroughly and gently, between the teeth and under the gums.
2. Brush each side of every tooth as well as the gums.
3. Clean the tongue by using a tongue cleaner or brush, especially the back of the tongue.

Between meals, rinse with water, chew sugarless gum, or eat an apple, celery, or carrots.

14

FEAR AND ANXIETY OF DENTAL TREATMENT

Conquering the Abyss

Fear is only as deep as the mind allows.
—*Japanese Proverb*

Fibromyalgia is a condition in which you may have to live with daily pain. Not surprisingly, depression often accompanies fibromyalgia as well, along with the stress of coping with a disorder that often makes even routine chores unbearable. Other real-life concerns such as relationships, the future, and finances may place a strain on not just the heart and other organs, but also on dental health. As we've noted often in the previous chapters, it is always best to seek out professional care before dental problems become serious. Some people find it frightening and difficult to follow that sound advice.

Past experiences and emotions often keep people from seeking needed dental treatment. Their reticence may lead to extensive dental deterioration that eventually affects the whole body and worsens symptoms of fibromyalgia. Estimates suggest that almost fifty percent of Americans avoid preventive dental care because of fear and anxiety. If you're fearful of the dentist's office, it doesn't really matter whether the ultimate source of your stress and anxiety is related to your fibromyalgia or you simply share an aversion to dental care with millions of other people who don't have fibromyalgia. Either way, avoiding necessary dental care can make your life even more complicated. You need some healthy coping strategies to overcome your fears. That's the purpose of this chapter.

How Did This Start, and What Do I Do Now?

No one knows the exact cause of fear and anxiety before dental appointments, but many dental phobias seem to go back to a specific memory of a childhood experience with a dentist or a negative experience recounted by someone else, such as a parent's often-told and increasingly elaborated dental office horror story. Patients have told me that they remember how frightened they were in early childhood by the high-pitched whine of dental drills, or by seeing a Novocain syringe. Many people get a little wobbly just glancing at a tray of cleaning instruments or a dot of blood on a piece of gauze. Let's face it: many people are just plain squeamish in a medical or dental setting and their early memories reinforce their anxiety.

Dealing with the Fear

Dentists are very much aware that many of their patients suffer from some form of anxiety or fear when they arrive for an appointment. There are many ways to get help from your dentist for dental anxiety and fear. Begin by finding a dentist with whom you can communicate and feel comfortable. You should feel very comfortable discussing your concerns about your treatment and fears associated with your appointment. At times, just a better understanding and knowledge of the treatment you're about to receive will help alleviate stress and anxiety. It's often the fear of the unknown that heightens tension. Discussing any doubts about what is going to happen and asking for help during a dental visit can make the visit more enjoyable and easier. This will take some effort on your part. It will be teamwork between you and the dental staff.

Research shows us that not only do stress and anxiety affect the health of the body, they also adversely affect the decision to seek dental treatment. You should understand that when you are relaxed and comfortable during your dental visit, the dentist can provide better care. If he is constantly concentrating on keeping you calm and relaxed, it makes it difficult for him to concentrate on the technique he is performing in your mouth. However, clinical professionals realize that patients have a right to voice their concerns to their physician or dentist.

For example, if you feel that lengthy appointments exacerbate fibromyalgia symptoms for you, ask the dentist for shorter appointments. If you still have good days and some bad days, you may want to ask your dentist to put you on a short call list, so when they have an opening they will call to offer you the option of coming in. If you are having a good day, you can go in for treatment; otherwise you can ask to be called another day. This way, you won't be taking valuable appointment time away from the dentist because you didn't show up when he was expecting you. Communicating this and working out a system with your dentist will help you complete your dental treatment, and make it easier for the dentist to provide the best care possible for you.

There are many ways to help with dental fear and anxiety. The more you get involved and take charge of your fear, the better the results will be. The following are some techniques that might help:

◆ On the day of your appointment, avoid caffeine for at least six hours prior to your visit. If you are keyed up to begin with, caffeine will only heighten your anxiety. Sugary foods will also increase your anxiety. Instead, opt for a high protein snack or meal before you head to the dental office. This will actually calm you. Sip on calming chamomile tea on your way to the appointment or in the waiting room.

◆ Practice slow and focused breathing. People who are anxious tend to hold their breath. Deep, slow breathing has calming qualities. The more oxygen you have available, the less panic you will feel.

◆ If your dentist doesn't provide CDs or audiotapes to listen to, take your own portable player and listen to your favorite CD, audiotape, or radio program.

◆ Another comforting technique to practice in the dental chair is daydreaming. Hold nothing back from your imagination. Dream about beautiful places where you would rather be or make plans about the weekend or the holidays. Let your mind wander far and wide, but keep your thoughts pleasant. Visualize how healthy and beautiful your teeth are going to be after the treatment, and how easily the work will be accomplished. Your efforts at mind-over-matter will provide you with a powerful coping mechanism and will get easier with practice.

◆ Before your dentist gets started, ask any questions you wish about the treatment you're about to receive and make sure you're comfortable about your appointment. Work out a hand signal to let the dentist know if you want a break or if you feel pain.

◆ Your dentist can also prescribe anti-anxiety medication such as Valium or give you **nitrous oxide** (**laughing gas**) to help you relax. (Nitrous oxide is not for everyone, and it has an opposite effect on some, making them feel more nervous.)

◆ **General anesthesia** is another method to manage stress, fear, and anxiety for those who have a phobia about dental treatment. Many dental offices have a general anesthesiologist to provide this service to their patients. The presence of that professional specialist makes anesthesia much safer than having the dentist administer general anesthesia while performing dentistry. The anesthesiologist can monitor your heart rate and other vital signs while the dentist is providing the dental treatment. It's best to get as much of the treatment as possible in one appointment, while under general anesthesia.

♦ Some dentists help their patients relax by creating a calming office atmosphere. The dental "spa" has become popular across the United States as dentists offer dental chairs that massage their patients or apply acupressure and massages on their feet during the dental appointment. The atmosphere of the dental office certainly will make a difference in helping you to relax.

Hope for the Truly Phobic

Many people feel a bit anxious before a dental appointment; some people are seriously frightened. They can't sleep for a week; just the thought of the dental visit raises their blood pressure and makes them feel ill. They try to avoid the situation at all cost. This kind of behavior describes a person who has a "phobia," an irrational fear of a situation, activity, or object. People with a phobia about a dental visit will avoid the situation and repeatedly make and break appointments. As soon as they walk into a dental office, they feel panicky. Their hearts begin to beat faster. Their palms sweat and they feel shortness of breath.

If you know that you need dental treatment desperately, but suffer from severe phobia that is preventing you from getting help, it may be time to seek a psychiatrist or psychologist for help or to find a dentist who administers general anesthesia in the office. With general anesthesia, you arrive in the office with a companion. The anesthesia is administered through the arm and next thing you know it's all over and you're going home. This is an excellent option and all you have to do is get to the office. You could also ask your physician or dentist to prescribe an anti-anxiety or sleeping medication for you to take the night before your appointment.

Unfortunately, if the phobia remains unresolved, once the painful teeth are treated under general anesthesia, many people will return to their phobic feelings and avoid further dental work. By not going back to the dentist for preventive treatment, they're back to square one. They may have spent thousands of dollars for treatment that, for lack of simple preventive care, they may need again. There are several techniques that can be used to help with phobias. If you can handle the least threatening procedure at the dentist's office—a routine cleaning—use the appointment as an opportunity to practice techniques that you may find helpful in alleviating your phobia. Below are some methods that may help you with your phobia. Remember, though: You should consult with a therapist if you know in your heart that your phobia is clearly too difficult for you to handle by yourself.

- One of the most common relaxation techniques is **progressive muscle relaxation (PMR)**. It was first developed in the 1930s by Edmund Jacobson. The theory is that if you relax physically, you will relax mentally. Progressive muscle relaxation involves tensing and relaxing groups of muscles. The idea is that, with practice, you should be able to relax when you want to. To learn this technique you must practice it for about ten to twenty minutes a day. The first time you try it, it may take about an hour to go through the process. If you have any injuries, consult with your physician before starting. It has been suggested that it may take six to eight weeks before you notice a difference in your composure and control over phobias.
- **Autogenic relaxation** involves using imagery to relax. It provides a substitute for people who experience pain from the muscle tensing necessary for progressive muscle relaxation. Lie down or sit in a comfortable position in a quiet room. You will be using the same muscle groups as in progressive muscle relaxation, but the technique is different. You may want to imagine yourself surrounded by warm water or that you feel the warm sun and a gentle breeze on you as you're

Progressive Muscle Relaxation Exercise

You should sit in a quiet room without any disturbances whenever you practice progressive muscle relaxation. This will help you to concentrate physically and mentally. Sit in a comfortable chair with both feet on the floor or try lying flat on the floor. Use the position that feels the most comfortable. Begin by taking a deep breath and picture all the tension virtually leaving your body, moving through every single muscle starting with the top of your head all the way to the bottom of your feet. Next begin the exercise by tensing each muscle group and holding for about ten seconds or as long as you can take it, followed by relaxing it.

1. Right hand and forearm
   Make a fist.
   Release.
2. Right upper arm.
   Bend the arm and feel the tenseness move to your biceps and
      shoulder.
   Release and let the right arm go limp. Feel the warmth and let
      it go.
3. Left hand and forearm.
   Make a fist.
   Release.
4. Left upper arm.
   Bend the arm and tighten the muscles all the way up to the
      biceps and shoulder.
   Release and let the arm go limp.
5. Forehead: Frown as hard as you can.
   Raise your eyebrows as high as you can.
   Relax your face.

6. Eyes and cheeks.

   Squeeze the eyes.

   Relax.

7. Shoulder and neck.

   Shrug your shoulders as high as you can and then relax them. Pull your lips sideways as wide as you can, tensing the front of your neck as well. Relax the lips and neck.

8. Chest and back.

   Breathe in deeply and hold your breath, pressing the shoulders together at the back at the same time.

   Let your shoulders hang; breathe normally.

9. Belly.

   Tighten the abdominal muscles (or draw in the belly).

   Release.

10. Right thigh.

   Tense these muscles and then relax.

   Release.

11. Right calf.

   Lift up the right heel (be careful not to cramp).

   Release.

12. Right foot.

   Point the toes.

   Release.

13. Left thigh.

   Tense the muscles.

   Relax.

14. Left calf.

   Lift up the left heel.

   Release.

15. Left foot.

   Point the toes. Release.

With practice, you should be able to perform this technique with your eyes shut. I have actually walked my patients through a shortened form of this technique while they sat in the dental chair. You can do this by yourself, or ask your dentist to help you. In the abbreviated dental chair technique, I have my patient concentrate on tensing and relaxing muscle groups starting with the top of the head, to the neck and moving down to the shoulders, arms, hands, legs, and feet. This technique is much more effective if the person has been practicing it for several weeks on a daily basis. Take your time and enjoy the process. When you're done, just sit or lie there and feel the relaxation, along with taking some deep breaths.

following the steps below. See yourself in a field filled with beautiful flowers and grass. You can also enhance the experience by practicing biofeedback phrases such as "I feel so peaceful and relaxed" or "My mind and body are at peace." A great opportunity to practice this technique is at bedtime, especially if you are among those who have fibromyalgia and have difficulty falling asleep.

1. Take some deep breaths and close your eyes. With each exhalation, feel yourself becoming more relaxed.
2. Starting with the head and face, tell yourself that these muscles are getting very heavy and relaxed and all the tension is totally leaving them. Picture this with your mind.
3. Move to the shoulder and neck area and repeat by visualizing all the tension leaving the muscles and they are getting more and more relaxed.
4. Move to the chest, abdomen, and lower back.
5. Next move to the arms and hands.
6. End with the legs and feet.

♦ Other forms of treatment for phobias include exposing your-self to the situation that is the perceived cause of phobia. This technique is known as **desensitizing therapy**. For example, make routine check-up and cleaning appointments three to six months ahead. As you keep these minor appoint-ments, you will learn to be more relaxed should you need other types of treatment. Keeping regular dental check-up appointments will also prevent minor situations from turning into advanced problems.

In summary, don't allow anxiety, stress, or phobias to stand in the way of seeking needed dental treatment. Take action, one sim-ple step at a time, such as trying some of the exercises recom-mended in this chapter. Break the cycle by doing something different and moving in a positive direction. Don't allow negative things about yourself to take control and force you to react in self-defeating ways. Consciously and confidently taking a first step toward change will be the most important thing you can do and will, once again, give you added confidence to deal with the chal-lenges fibromyalgia presents.

15

FINDING A DENTIST

How to Find the Needle in the Haystack

Are you one of those people who refuses to get needed dental treatment because you just can't find a "good" dentist? Have you gone from one dentist to another and still have not found the one who you feel really "cares" about you? Finding the right dentist for you takes more than looking in the yellow pages and pointing to the first large ad that you see. Just what determines the qualities of the "right" dentist—their education, how long they've been in practice, or how their office looks?

An important part of finding a dentist, or any other kind of healthcare practitioner, is the matter of personal "fit." A friend or relative may have found "the best dentist in the world," while you may simply not warm up to that person. As the Italians say, you're not "simpatico." For example, if you are an introvert and your dentist is a talker who likes to excitedly discuss his golf game and how each player on the local baseball team scores hits, it may appear that he or she is more concerned about these matters than you and your oral care. But your friend or relative who is an extrovert and enjoys sports might think that same person is the best dentist they've ever had—irrespective of skill and training—just because they relate on similar topics and tastes.

Having similar personalities is important in choosing a dentist; however, there are other important factors that you should also consider.

Location, Location, Location

How convenient is it to see this dentist? A dental practice located within a five to ten mile radius of your home is reasonable. This is important because with your fibromyalgia-related fatigue you don't necessarily like driving long distances. Distance is especially important if you have an emergency, because you'll want to be able to see that dentist as soon as possible. If you need to make appointments based on short notice, living close by makes it easier to do so.

Appointment Availability

If appointments with a dentist aren't available for one or more months, this is not the dental office for you. Limited availability may indicate that the office is very busy and the staff may be overbooked or they have limited days or hours when they see patients. Dentists with a well-managed practice know what their limits are and avoid getting stretched so far that they can't render quality treatment.

It's easy for a dentist to overdo it by overbooking patients, being open six to seven days a week with long hours, and providing most of the treatment without help from associates. Dentistry is a very demanding profession. Not only must dentists provide precise treatment that requires concentration, but daily business activities also take time and energy.

Another appointment practice to be aware of, given your fibromyalgia, is the dental practice's policy on missed appointments.

Naturally you should show up for appointments if possible, but you don't want to be charged for a broken appointment (which some offices do) if you wake up on the day of your dental visit with pain and are just having a very bad day or because you've suffered a memory lapse and completely forgotten your appointment. ("Fibro-fog" strikes again!) If the dentist understands fibromyalgia, he or she will be able to accommodate appointments for you on short notice when you are having a "good day."

Services Offered

Dentists need to keep up with new research and new materials in order to give you proper information and provide treatment options to solve your oral care problems. Every two years, all dentists must renew their licenses. This requires fifty hours of continuing education. However, some dentists still only offer one form of dental filling—the amalgam or silver mercury type—even though studies have shown that newer forms of white restorations are very durable. Furthermore, these white "composite" fillings are technique-sensitive and must be placed precisely or they may fail. It takes time, training, and money to reorient an existing practice that is used to amalgam fillings and switch to white fillings.

Another example of keeping up-to-date is a dentist's use of a non-surgical gum treatment versus the traditional surgical therapy. Some dentists may not want to take the time to learn the new techniques of non-surgical gum treatments and refer you for surgery at the first sign of gum disease. Learning new techniques and incorporating them into practice is time-consuming and costly and some dentists may not be willing to take the trouble. A dentist who offers general dentistry should offer all forms of filling material options, crowns, bridges and dentures, TMJ therapy and gum treatments. However, there are certain disciplines, such as implants, gum surgery, and difficult root canals that should be referred to a specialist, although many general dentists have chosen to seek extensive training in these areas and do successfully perform them.

Communication Skills of the Dentist

Some dentists want patients to come to their offices and accept whatever treatment plan they offer without any explanation of what caused their dental problem and what options are available for treatment. That's probably not the style you're looking for because you want to know that the dentist cares about your individual needs. Fibromyalgia is a disorder that requires T.L.C. from the dentist during treatment or stress, anxiety, and pain may make your symptoms worse. Fear of a dental visit is mostly caused by fear of the unknown. If you are comfortable asking your dentist questions until you understand what caused your problem and what the treatment options are, that's probably the dentist for you.

On the other hand, in defense of the dentist, I encourage you not to arrive for every appointment with a notebook of 100 questions you expect the dentist to answer. The dentist's time should also be respected. The time to discuss all your concerns should be during the initial examination. As the dentist completes the examination, try to ask as many of your questions as possible. This doesn't mean that you shouldn't ask any questions or discuss your concerns during subsequent appointments, but please be considerate of the dentist's time constraints as well. If you find a dentist with whom you feel comfortable, your questions and concerns will probably be covered during the initial examination.

The Staff

A well-managed dental practice has well-chosen and well-trained staff who care about you as much as the dentist does. From your

---

How to have stress free dental appointments:

From the very beginning of your relationship, you can make interactions with your dentist stress-free by employing a number of these techniques:

- Explain to your chosen dentist your fibromyalgia-related problems (or show your dentist this book). Ask not to be charged for breaking appointments if you are too sick to keep your appointment.
- Ask to be on a short call list. When you are having a good day, you can call and be seen that day.
- Ask that your appointments be kept short.

Let your dentist know how you will communicate with signals if you should need a break.

---

first contact, everyone from the receptionist to the dental assistants, hygienist, and associate dentist(s), should treat you with respect and give you the impression that they are there for you. If you see signs of ill feelings between staff, gossiping, and inappropriate behavior, this may be a sign of stress in that office, which may reflect on your treatment.

Cleanliness

I remember when I began practicing dentistry in the 1970s that we didn't use dental gloves during treatment. We washed our hands and launched into treatment on our patients. The only time we used gloves was during oral surgery. Today, times have changed and with the onset of concerns about HIV/AIDS not only are all dentists and assistants required to use gloves, but also masks and gowns, and to take other precautions. Sterilization requirements have also changed. Some dentists are more meticulous about sterilization than others. When you walk into an office, you should get an impression of how demanding the dentist is regarding sterilization and cleanliness, especially in the treatment rooms. Don't be afraid to ask the dentist what the practice's sterilization standards are. The Occupational Safety and Health Administration (OSHA) and the American Dental Association (ADA) have set strict standards and guidelines on how sterilization should be carried out in dental offices. Disposables should be used for many purposes. Any object that is handled during treatment must be covered with a disposable sheet. This includes the switch and handles for overhead patient lights, the switch that makes the dental chair recline or rise, and the headrest of the dental chair. All counters must be wiped carefully with disinfectant after each patient visit. All instruments should be brought into the room in sterilized bags and opened as the dentist begins treatment. This should include the dental drill and "burs" used in the dental drill to clean and shape teeth for restorations. Again, years ago this was not the protocol. Just wiping the drill with a disinfectant was satisfactory. Today, they must be properly sterilized. There are different methods of sterilization. Most dentists use one of the following:

1. Chemical vapor **autoclave**
2. Steam autoclave
3. Dry heat oven

Trays that hold instruments must also be covered by disposables. Although it is very rare indeed that contagious diseases are acquired in the dental office, it is important for the dentist to provide dental care in a properly sterilized environment, for the health of the patient and the staff.

Education and Training Background

The United States has excellent dental schools that provide top training for dentists. Even foreign graduates who wish to practice here must first take an examination, followed by two years of further education in an accredited dental school in the United States, followed by national and state examinations for licensing. However, if you want to know, don't be embarrassed to ask what dental school the dentist attended, his or her year of graduation, and any other pertinent educational experience the dentist has pursued. If you're too embarrassed to ask the dentist, there is another option. Every dentist is regulated through the state's licensing board. You can either visit their Web site or locate their telephone number through the American Dental Association (800-621-8099). The Web site for the American Dental Association is www.ada.org. The Web site of your state's dental board can be found by entering "Dental Board of (name of state)" in the search engine. Once the Web site is found, there are options to click on how to get information about a licensed dentist in that state. Complaints against a dentist can also be filed through the dental board of your state.

Both the American Dental Association and your local dental board web site offer other helpful information to consumers such as how to avoid quacks and specific accreditation needed to be a dentist.

Insurance and Financial Options

It is obviously desirable to find a dentist who accepts your insurance plan, but this should not be a priority in choosing a dentist. In defense of many dentists who don't accept any insurance plans, this practice could be due to the demands many insurance companies place on dentists to view their patients in an excessively commercial way. This is especially true of the **HMO** plans that demand numerous forms to be filled out and filed, and that every "i" be dotted and every "t" crossed to prevent lawsuits for their companies. Excessive insurance paperwork can force dental offices to hire more staff just to handle the paper trail and to see more patients to be able to make a profit.

With some HMO dental plans, you are normally assigned to a specific dental office or choose from a list of offices that have a contract with the HMO. You can only change to another office once a year, unless you request a change due to some specific pre-set guidelines. With a **PPO** type of plan, you may go to any dentist on the insurance company's list. With PPO insurance, you may change dentists when you wish without any explanations or requests to the insurance company, as long as the new dentist has a contract with that particular plan. With most PPOs, you may go to an outside non-contracted dentist, but you may have to pay a slight out-of-pocket amount on top of what the insurance company will pay the dentist. Many offices also offer financing, with interest-free payments. If that is important to you, then you should choose a dentist that offers that option as well.

Putting It All Together

Unfortunately there are no dentists who specialize in fibromyalgia and the special concerns you are facing. Just where do you find a dentist that has all the qualities you need? Here are some suggestions:

◆ Start by asking friends, relatives, and coworkers for referrals to their dentists. Remember, just because that dentist worked well with your friend, relative, or coworker doesn't mean they will work well with you. The other choices are the yellow pages and the local dental societies.

- Once you have a list of dentists, call their offices. Your first impression about the office begins with the receptionist. If the receptionist is willing and trained to answer questions and you like what you hear, make an appointment to go for either an examination or just a consultation. If you don't want to take the plunge and make a first appointment yet, you could also ask the receptionist if you could just come and visit and possibly meet the dentist or pick up any brochures they may have. This visit may give you valuable information about the office in general. Usually, first impressions give good insight into the overall picture.
- If you are on the guaifenesin protocol, discuss your concerns with the dentist to make sure he or she is willing to work with you on this issue.
- Once you've chosen a dentist and go for the appointment, begin with a minor treatment, unless you feel very good about the dentist and the office as a whole or need treatment as soon as possible. People have contacted me from many parts of the country and asked me to provide referrals because they could not decide on dentists. In these cases, I recommend that they find a dentist for now, just to take care of the needed care, and keep looking for the dentist they finally want to work with for more extensive treatment.

Once you've found the dentist of your dreams, complete your treatment and keep up with your regular check-ups and cleanings. Don't allow fear, money, lack of time, or any other reason keep you from completing your treatment. If money is an issue, you'd be surprised if you really consider it, how much money you waste on things that don't matter, such as daily exotic coffee drinks at three to five dollars each, candy and junk food, clothing that you may wear once and hang in your closet never to be worn again, and other useless things. If illness, such as fibromyalgia is a problem, see the dentist on "good days."

Questions to Ask the Dentist You Are Interviewing

1. Which dental school did you attend?
2. How long have you been practicing dentistry?
3. What are your office hours?
4. How are emergencies handled?
5. How are financial matters handled? Do you accept any insurance? Do you have payment plans?
6. Do you have any understanding of fibromyalgia?
7. Do you treat TMJ?
8. What other services do you offer?
9. What types of filling materials do you offer?
10. How far in advance can I schedule my first appointment?
11. What are your office hours?

Observations Made After the Interview

1. Were you treated courteously or indifferently, either on the phone or when you arrived at the office?
2. Was the staff friendly and responsive, or distant and curt?
3. How long did you have to wait in the waiting room before being seen? Emergencies happen with other patients that may delay your appointment. However, ultimately the dentist affects appointment punctuality.
4. Does the office appear clean and tidy or dirty, dusty, and cluttered?
5. When you meet the doctor, does he or she listen and hear you and respond with compassion and knowledge?
6. Is the dentist responsive to your concerns and willing to take the time to understand more about fibromyalgia and the special concerns that apply to you?

In summary, if you need immediate care, find a dentist as quickly as you can to treat that condition. Otherwise, find a dentist who matches all your requirements. Remember, you are choosing someone to whom you will entrust your oral health and care, so take your time and choose wisely.

A word of caution for those seeking a "holistic dentist." Holistic dentists have been trained at the dental schools that all other dentists in your communities have been trained in. The only difference is that the holistic dentist offers other forms of dental treatments that have not been approved by the F.D.A. or the mainstream dental community and the organization that represents mainstream dentistry, the American Dental Association. When I get e-mails and telephone calls requesting referrals to holistic dentists, I advise people to find a dentist who meets the criteria I have listed in this chapter, not to seek a holistic dentist who might cure fibromyalgia with the removal of mercury silver fillings. What is most important is the professional bond you form with your dentist so together you can bring optimum health to this very important organ we call the oral cavity. As a result, you will be checking off one more items on your inventory list toward management of fibromyalgia symptoms.

16

FLUORIDE,
FOR BETTER OR FOR WORSE

What You Need to Know

The only way to keep your health is to eat what you don't want,
drink what you don't like, and do what you'd rather not.
—*Mark Twain*

Who would have imagined that adding a naturally occurring mineral—fluoride—to the water supply would have stirred such heated controversy in communities throughout America? Most of the dispute has been about water fluoridation and not as much about fluoride as an ingredient in dental products. Groups have blamed fluoridation for everything from cancer to usurping our freedom of choice. Is there a final answer to the fluoride controversy that resolves whether it is an evil conspiracy or a God-sent prevention of tooth decay?

Fluoride is a form of the naturally occurring element, fluorine, found in the earth's crust. Fluoride is a negatively charged "ion" and must combine with positive ions such as calcium or sodium to form stable compounds that we know of as **calcium fluoride** or sodium fluoride. These forms of fluoride are found in the ocean, air and in many foods, especially in teas and ocean fish.

The fluoride controversy has been ongoing ever since its effect on tooth decay was discovered in the 1940s. It was quite by accident that the decay-preventive role of fluoride became known at that time. Dentists became aware that in some communities, concentrations of naturally occurring fluoride (calcium fluoride) in the water supply had "mottled" the teeth of many of its residents. The mottled appearance or "enamel fluorosis" formed chalklike markings across the tooth's surface. Notably, it turned out that the people in these communities had less decay in their teeth than in other communities.

This observation led to studies on the affect of fluoride on teeth. There has been an overwhelming amount of research on the subject, which has generally concluded that an optimal concentration of fluoride in a community's drinking water inhibits dental **caries**. Nevertheless, the fluoride controversy has persisted over the years and fluoridation continues to be accused of causing cancer, bone fractures, and other health hazards.

As you'll learn in this chapter, fluoride is clearly useful in preventing tooth decay and treating sensitive teeth. These issues can be especially important for fibromyalgia sufferers, so this chapter should be particularly pertinent to you. And in general, because fluoride use is so widespread and so controversial, knowing more about it will make you a well informed consumer. Be aware, though, that while fluoride offers benefits, and while research has rejected the notion that it causes either cancer or fractures, too much fluoride can be hazardous.

How Does Fluoride Prevent Cavities?

Tooth decay results from demineralization or loss of minerals from the tooth surface. Studies have concluded that these demineralized tooth surfaces have become re-mineralized with the aid of fluorides. The re-mineralization strengthens the enamel crystals (hydroxyapatite) and makes the tooth more resistant to attack by acid in the mouth. In other words, fluoride makes teeth harder. Demineralized areas of teeth have a whitish appearance, and are not visible under X-ray. Because these areas are not detected at routine dental check-ups and re-mineralization is possible, fluoride treatments are recommended by dentists twice a year for children as a way to prevent cavities. Adults can also benefit from weekly or daily at-home fluoride applications as we'll discuss later in the chapter.

Using Fluoride to Prevent Cavities

The easiest and least expensive way to prevent decay with fluoride is by adding it to tap water, but most of the controversy regarding fluoride revolves around that very practice. Studies have concluded that the approximate optimal amount of fluoride in water to help reduce dental caries and minimize the risk of **dental fluorosis** is one part per million (PPM). A call to your local community water supplier will let you know if your water is fluoridated and if so, at what concentration. You can also check this information on the Internet through the Centers for Disease Control and Prevention (www.cdc.gov/oralhealth/data_systems/index.htm).

States that currently fluoridate water supplies include: Arizona, Colorado, Delaware, Florida, Georgia, Illinois, Indiana, Iowa, Maine, Massachusetts, Michigan, Minnesota, Nebraska, New Hampshire, Nevada, North Dakota, Oklahoma, Pennsylvania, and Wisconsin.

Approximately sixty percent of community water supplies in the United States contain fluoride in concentrations from 0.7 to 1.2 parts per million (0.7–1.2 milligrams per liter). However, many people don't drink tap water but prefer bottled water. Current FDA regulations require fluoridated bottled water to be labeled as such. Most bottled water marketed in the United States contains less than 0.3 PPM fluoride, although some brands contain the "optimal" concentration of approximately 1.0 PPM.

Brushing with **fluoride toothpaste** is another way to affect demineralized enamel in teeth. In the United States, fluoride concentration in toothpaste is 1,000–1,100 PPM. Although it can help avoid tooth decay, fluoride toothpaste contributes to the risk of enamel fluorosis in children because the swallowing reflex of children younger than six years old is not always well controlled. A child-sized toothbrush covered with a full strip of toothpaste holds approximately 0.75–1.0 grams of toothpaste, and each gram of fluoride toothpaste in the United States contains approximately 1.0 milligram of fluoride. Children can inadvertently swallow as much as 0.8 gram, especially if the toothpaste looks appealing and similar to candy. As a result, multiple brushings with fluoride toothpaste each day can result in ingestion of excess fluoride. This may not only result in dental fluorosis but in other serious health problems and can be fatal.

Ingestion of high doses of fluoride can be toxic. One study determined the toxic dose of fluoride to be five milligrams per kilogram. All toothpastes sold in the United States that contain fluoride are required to warn parents to keep it out of the hands of children and to call a poison control center if large amounts are ingested. The American Dental Association (**ADA**) has said this warning is "unnecessary."

Signs and symptoms of acute fluoride poisoning include:

◆ Nausea
◆ Vomiting
◆ Abdominal pain
◆ Increased salivation
◆ Watery eyes
◆ Shallow breathing
◆ Convulsions
◆ Diarrhea
◆ Cramps
◆ Cardiac arrhythmia
◆ Coma

Fluoride may present a risk if a person ingests it from multiple sources, for example from the water supply, in supplements, toothpaste, and food. You should evaluate all these factors before adding fluoride treatments and supplements.

Fluoride mouth rinse is another means of delivering concentrated fluoride to the teeth. For effective decay prevention in adults, daily rinses (0.05 sodium fluoride, obtained over-the-counter) and weekly rinses (0.02 sodium fluoride, obtained by prescription) could be used. However, it is important to understand that without proper brushing, flossing and regular professional dental cleanings, fluoride rinses are not as beneficial.

Mouth rinse products present some risks for children. Studies have indicated that some young children might swallow substantial amounts of fluoride mouth rinse, especially if they are attracted to the color or taste. Also, it is extremely important to not have children rinse with any mouthwash containing alcohol.

Dietary Fluoride Supplements

Tablets, lozenges, or liquids containing sodium fluoride as the active ingredient have been used since the 1940s. They are supplied with either 1.0, 0.5, or 0.25 milligram fluoride. The purpose of supplements is mostly for areas where drinking water is not fluoridated. Studies have shown that fluoride supplements taken by infants and children before their teeth erupt reduce the prevalence and severity of cavities.

Fluoride supplements should not be taken in communities where fluoridated water content is greater than 0.6 parts per million (0.6 milligrams per liter).

Fluoride Gels Applied by the Dentist

High concentrations of fluoride compounds are sometimes applied directly to patients' teeth during dental visits. Gels are usually applied through a mouth tray and contain 1.23 percent acidulated phosphate fluoride (APF). Clinical trials conducted from 1940–1970 demonstrated that professionally applied fluorides effectively reduce cavities in children. Tray-type fluoride treatments are especially important to prevent decay in people undergoing radiation or chemotherapy.

Fluoride and Sensitive Teeth

There are various causes for sensitive teeth and your dentist can determine the reason for the problem. If the sensitivity is caused by receded gums that expose the root surface of the tooth, your dentist may prescribe an over-the-counter fluoride gel (usually 0.4 percent stannous fluoride) or desensitizing toothpaste that contains either potassium nitrate or strontium chloride. These ingredients help block transmission of sensation from the tooth to the nerve, but they may cause sores in the mouth due to an allergic reaction. This is important for those with numerous chemical sensitivities, which is not uncommon among people with fibromyalgia.

Sensitive teeth are very common for individuals living with fibromyalgia. Either prescribed or over-the-counter fluoride gel brushed or rubbed on the gums and other sensitive areas is helpful. Relief may not be noticed immediately and may take as long as a month to be noticed. For those on the guaifenesin program of Dr. Paul St. Amand (discussed in Chapter Four), it is of course important to choose a fluoride gel that has no mint or other salicylates.

Applying fluoride gel at bedtime, either daily or two to three times a week, depending on the level of sensitivity, should provide relief. If this treatment doesn't help, your dentist can place a bonded composite material in the area. This will cover the exposed root surface, protect it from sensitivity due to cold, and protect it against further wear from routine brushing.

Cancer, Bone Fractures, and Other Claims Against Fluoride

The National Cancer Institute has concluded, based on studies produced over the last forty years, that fluoride in drinking water does not pose any detectable cancer risk to humans. Bone fractures due to fluoride (**skeletal fluorosis**) have been documented in women who were receiving forty to sixty milligrams of fluoride daily for eleven to twenty-one months. The conclusion from these studies was that kidney problems and renal insufficiency were the root cause, and these disorders, in turn, caused excessive fluoride retention.

The only two documented hazards directly attributable to fluoride are dental mottling brought about by excessive fluoride intake, and fluoride poisoning due to ingestion of toxic levels of fluoride.

Finding the Correct Fluoride Dose

Fluoride, in appropriate doses, has been shown to prevent cavities and help protect teeth from attack by acid produced by bacteria.

The Food and Nutrition Board of the Institute of Medicine of the U.S. National Academy of Sciences has recommended the following adequate intakes for fluoride:

Infants
0–6 months	0.01 mg/day
7–12 months	0.5 mg/day

Children
1–3 years	0.7 mg/day
4–8 years	1 mg/day
9–13 years	2 mg/day
14–18 years	3 mg/day

Adults
Males 19 and over	4 mg/day
Females 19 and over	3 mg/day

Pregnancy and
Breastfeeding	3 mg/day

This is true for children as well as adults. However, **dental fluorosis** in children and **skeletal fluorosis** in children and adults may occur with excessive intake of fluoride. It is important to determine the amount of fluoride taken from water supply, before beginning the use of other forms of fluoride. Remember that fluoride can come from the water supply, from toothpaste, from foods and processed beverages, and from various fluoride treatments. Recommended adequate intake of fluoride for adults is between three (women) to four (men) milligrams daily. Excessive doses can be harmful; in fact, a single oral dose of five to ten grams of sodium fluoride may be lethal.

Different Forms of Fluoride and Their Uses

Here are the different forms of fluoride. Choose the one that best suits your health and dental situation.

- *Fluoride* is a trace mineral and is also known as fluorine. It's found in nature, but never alone, because it is a reactive element. When added to water or dental products, it must be in compound form.
- *Calcium fluoride* (CaF_2), also known as fluorite or fluorspar, is a naturally occurring mineral and the type found in natural fluoridated water. It is nearly insoluble and cannot be easily absorbed by the body.
- *Stannous fluoride* is a compounded form of fluorine used to fluoridate toothpaste and mouth rinse. One percent stannous fluoride contains approximately 0.25 percent fluoride. When provided in concentrated gel form, stannous flouride aids in preventing cavities on roots of teeth with receded gums. This form is also ideal for treating sensitivity in these areas. Stannous fluoride may etch composites and porcelain fillings and crowns.

+ **Sodium fluoride** is also commonly used as a cavity-fighting agent in commercial toothpastes, although it didn't make its commercial debut until 1982. It works well with the kinds of silica abrasives used as polishing agents in translucent gel toothpastes. Sodium fluoride is a close chemical relative of sodium chloride, or ordinary table salt. Products containing one percent sodium fluoride contain approximately 0.50 percent fluoride. When recommended in concentrated gel form, it is ideal for acid-intolerant individuals such as those with reduced levels of saliva from chemotherapy and radiation therapy. Sodium fluoride does not etch dental work and is gentle on crowns and composites.

+ **Sodium monofluorophosphate (MFP)**—One percent sodium monofluorophosphate contains approximately 0.125 percent fluoride. It is used mostly in over-the-counter toothpaste and mouthwash.

  Note: The FDA (US Food and Drug Administration) has approved stannous fluoride, sodium fluoride, and sodium monofluorophosphate as the only forms of fluoride acceptable in toothpaste. All are derived from hydrofluoric acid, which in turn is made by reacting sulfuric acid with fluorspar, a calcium fluoride-rich ore.

+ **APF (acidulated phosphate fluoride)** is compounded from sodium fluoride and hydrofluoric acid. It is used in the prevention of dental caries, mostly in the dental office, where it is loaded in trays and left in the mouth for approximately one minute. One percent APF contains 1.0 percent fluoride.

+ **Fluorosilicic acid** is a chemical produced by phosphoric acid plants, which process phosphate rock into phosphoric acid. It is commonly used to fluoridate public water supplies. The chart below shows fluoridation examples in the Northwest and throughout the U.S. as was published in:

  http://www.ci.beaverton.or.us/departments/engineering/ eng_fluoridation.html

FLUORIDATION EXAMPLES IN THE NORTHWEST
AND THROUGHOUT THE U.S.

Water System	Population Served	Fluoride Dose (Target) mg/L	Chemical	Purity of Chemical[1]
Seattle Public Utilities	1,281,000	1.0	Fluorosilicic Acid	AWWA B703
Tacoma Water	316,850	1.0	Fluorosilicic Acid	AWWA B703
Everett, City of	96,000	1.0	Fluorosilicic Acid	AWWA B703
MWRA[2] (Boston)	2,200,000	1.0	Fluorosilicic Acid	AWWA B703
MWD[3]	18,000,000	0.7–0.8	Fluorosilicic Acid	AWWA B703
Chicago Dept. of Water	2,900,000	1.0	Fluorosilicic Acid	AWWA B703
Denver Water	1,081,000	0.9	Sodium Fluorosilicate	AWWA B702

1 Purity of Chemical is defined by applicable ANSI/AWWA specification.

2 Massachusetts Water Resources Authority.

3 Metropolitan Water District of Southern California.

17

ROOT CANAL THERAPY

What's Going On in There? Getting to the Root of It

Years ago, when a tooth became diseased or the **pulp** (soft, inner core of the tooth, which houses the nerve and blood supply) was injured, it was pulled. Today**, endodontic treatment** (root canal therapy) is a means of saving most teeth with a diseased or inflamed pulp. Tooth decay usually begins on a very small scale and spreads into the inner layers of the tooth. If a small cavity is ignored, it will continue to destroy tooth structure until it eventually causes inflammation or an infection of pulp tissue. At that stage, you may very well have moderate to severe pain and swelling. The tooth will require what's called "**root canal**" therapy or the alternative, which would be to pull the tooth.

This chapter will explain why root canal therapy is sometimes necessary and how it is performed. For the sake of completeness, we will also discuss some of the ideas of holistic dentistry about this subject, although I must stress that holistic theories are unproven and unsupported by research.

As with all of the other dental topics and procedures covered in this book, the needs of people with fibromyalgia remain in the forefront of my mind in this chapter. Root canal is undertaken because of a serious and potentially dangerous dental infection. It is unlikely that people with fibromyalgia are more prone to the need for root canal therapy than the general population, but failing to address the need for this treatment can have especially serious consequences for people with fibromyalgia. With this problem, as with all of the other forms of dental prevention and therapy, if you have fibromyalgia you must stay ahead of the potential serious consequences of dental neglect. If therapy is needed, get it promptly, but be a well-informed patient, too.

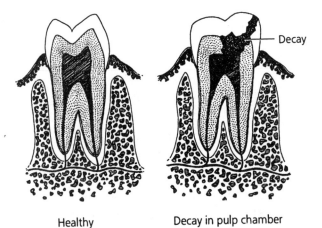

Healthy   Decay in pulp chamber

Figure 4

Each tooth has a central area called a "pulp," that extends the inner length of the tooth from the crown to the end of the root(s). Some teeth have only one root, while others, such as back teeth (**molars**), have two or three. The roots have "canals" that house the pulp tissue. This includes blood vessels, nerves and other tissue that carries nutrients to the tooth, and in baby (primary) teeth, helps them develop and grow. In the crown portion of each tooth, this pulp is protected by **dentin** and enamel that minimize any sensations such as cold or hot from being transmitted to the nerve as we eat or drink. An adult (permanent) tooth can survive without the pulp if it has to, because the tooth is fully developed and can get nourishment for stability from surrounding structures.

When the dentist tells you that a tooth requires root canal therapy, it is because this pulp tissue is either injured or infected. If there is an infection, then you may have to take antibiotics before the tooth is treated. Once a tooth infection sets in, if left untreated, it can spread and even cause serious illness. Sometimes a root canal is required owing to internal resorption, usually due to an immune system response to a tooth that has suffered trauma such as severe grinding, clenching or blow to the tooth.

The best way to prevent root canals is to seek dental treatment when problems first are noticed. For example, during routine six-month check-ups your dentist may notice a small area of decay starting in a tooth. If it is taken care of at this stage, it won't advance to damaging the nerve and requiring root canal.

I often hear patients talking about concerns of severe pain and discomfort during root canal procedure. Many have heard horror stories about intense pain and complications. However, those are only myths unless the person has waited until the infection has become very serious. Even then, once a qualified dentist determines treatment can be done and the tooth saved, the treatment should be no more painful then getting a tooth filled. Some cases may require two appointments to complete root canals. High-tech instruments in modern dentistry make root canals not only faster but also painless. Rotary instruments have been developed to start and finish the root canal with few chances for complications.

An **endodontist** is a dental specialist who only treats diseases involving pulp tissue, such as those requiring root canal therapy. Unless you are very anxious or have phobias about dental treatment, root canal therapy is usually done under local anesthetic. In simple terms, the treatment starts with the dentist making a very small opening on the crown of the tooth, and removes tooth structure down to the pulp.

The Root Canal Procedure

A rubber sheet (**rubber dam**) is used to isolate the tooth opening to the pulp tissue. Sensitive, small files are used to clean out the canals which house the nerve and blood supply. The area is irrigated and cleaned of all debris including infection. If the tooth is badly infected, a medication is inserted with a small piece of cotton over the area and the tooth is sealed with temporary cement. Antibiotics, anti-inflammatory and pain medication are prescribed and you are sent home. You return in about a week to finish the root canal. The area is cleaned and filed and filled with a biocompatible rubbery material called **gutta-percha**. This seals the canals and does not allow recontamination.

Root canal therapy is successful approximately ninety-five percent of the time. However, there are certain factors that can cause the tooth to need further surgery, re-treatment or even extraction. For example, if there is new decay due to poor hygiene, infection, or trauma to the tooth which results in a crack in the root, then further treatment may be necessary. If a tooth continues to be painful, it may mean there are other "accessory" small canals that were undetected, even with X-ray, and need to be cleaned and filled. Other complications may include breaking of the small sterile files into the canals. If this happens, the dentist or specialist may or may not be able to remove the broken instrument, depending on where it is in the canal.

Sometimes the tooth does not heal due to previous root fractures. In this case pain does not go away and the tooth may have to be pulled. Other complications may occur after the root canal is completed. A canal may become re-infected. In this case a procedure called "apicoectomy" is performed. With an **apicoectomy** or root-end resection, a small opening is made at the **apex** or tip of the root canal through the gums. The end of the root and the surrounding tissue are cleaned of any infection or inflammation and then sealed. This procedure is usually fifty percent successful. If pain returns, the tooth will have to be pulled.

Once the treatment is completed, a final **restoration** will be recommended. A **crown** is usually placed over a tooth that has had root canal therapy. If most of the tooth had to be cleaned out and removed, a "**post**" may also have to be placed to build a foundation for the crown.

Root Canals and Holistic Dentistry

Holistic dentists have raised some controversies about root canal therapy. Some holistic dentists and "biological dentists" claim that root canals should not be done at all and that teeth that have been root canalled should be pulled. They claim that the root canals create "focal points" that compromise the immune system and may be the source of illness. Many people with chronic illnesses like fibromyalgia are told that root canalled teeth should be pulled, even if there are no problems with them. A book with the title *Root Canal Cover-up* by George Meinig summarized all the controversy about root canals. The book focuses on the theme that "focal infections" in one area of the body (for example a tooth) may bring about disease in a totally different area or organ of the body (for example the heart).

This book is based on research done about 100 years ago by dentist Weston Price. Dr. Price took infected teeth from his patients who suffered from a wide range of serious "medical" problems. He implanted these under the skin of laboratory animals and discovered that the animals came down with the same illness as the person from whom the tooth was taken. He then planted healthy teeth of patients with the same disease in several lab animals and found they all came down with the same disease. For example, if the teeth came from individuals with infected kidneys, all the animals quickly developed infected kidneys! Dr. Price also claimed that most "focal infections" started with teeth and tonsils. He indicated the bacteria in infected teeth and tonsils mutate and become toxic, travel through the blood stream and lymphatic system to remote body parts causing disease. Dr. Price wrote that root canal treatment does not totally clear the infection in the teeth and "mutant" bacteria and toxins are still there and eventually spread to other organs.

What critics of this theory often ask is: if this important and very critical information is more than a theory, why hasn't it been found in other studies and brought into mainstream medicine? This question remains unanswered in the *Root Canal Cover-up* book.

Other holistic proponents feel root canals are acceptable, but that the canals should not be filled with the conventional gutta-percha material, which they call "toxic," but with a material called "Biocalex 6.9." Dental gutta-percha points are used to fill root canals and contain approximately nineteen to twenty-two percent gutta-percha (obtained from gutteferous trees), fifty-nine to seventy-five percent zinc oxide and other agents such as plastics, waxes, colors, metal sulfates, and resins. Both natural rubber latex and synthetic materials are used to manufacture gutta percha.

According to the American Association of Endodontists, gutta-percha has been used successfully for years as the filling materials for root canal therapy, because it is dimensionally stable, fills the root canal space without expanding, and is placed in conjunction with adhesive **cement** to ensure complete sealing of the root canal. Many journals have published reports concluding that this filling, which has been used for more than 100 years, is biocompatible and safe. However, if a person has latex allergies, the physician, patient and dentist should discuss the options and materials and techniques used for root canals. In 1999, Kleier and Shibilski reported in the *Journal of Endodontics* that they found no automatic cross-reactivity with gutta-percha in patients allergic to latex. They found that gutta-percha and natural rubber latex are significantly different. Other studies delineate the differences in chemical composition and manufacture between the two products and conclude that gutta-percha results in minimal reactions. In general, research indicates that if the gutta-percha is completely confined within the root canal space and encased in sealer, no antigen appears to react with the body's immune system. Other types of root canal material should be considered for those that are truly allergic and sensitive to latex of any kind. Those other options are "silver points" and pastes containing calcium hydroxide.

Biocalex 6.9 was originally marketed in France and introduced to the United States in 1995. It consists of heavy calcium oxide powder and liquid ethyl glycol. The dentist mixes the two ingredients and places the mixture in a moist canal. The American Association of Endodontists (AAE) indicates that the manufacturer cautions that the use of Biocalex in weakened roots may increase the risk of root fracture because the product expands six to nine times its original volume, and advises that zinc oxide should be added to the mixture in order to prevent expansion.

Besides Biocalex 6.9, holistic and biological dentists recommend treating root canals with "bio-frequencies." This is a very expensive treatment requiring several visits of fifty to one hundred dollars per session. The claim is that when a certain frequency is sent through the canals of teeth, bacteria, viruses, molds, fungus, candida, and parasites are destroyed. Once again, no research has been done that justifies this treatment. Another unproven holistic method for treating root canals entails use of a homeopathic product called Sanum Remedies. These remedies come from Germany and supposedly act as antibiotics and strengthen the immune system. However, even in Germany the use of this costly and unproven therapy is limited to holistic dentists. Conventional dentists use the same proven and carefully researched techniques around the world.

A Final Word of Warning

Many people erroneously feel that once the dentist prescribes antibiotics, they no longer will need the root canal treatment because the swelling and pain disappear. Unfortunately, the source of the infection, which is the decay in the tooth affecting the pulp tissue, is still present and bacteria will cause the swelling to return. Antibiotics only kill the bacteria temporarily. Because the source of infection remains present, the swelling will return and will usually be worse than before. Again, it is particularly dangerous for people with fibromyalgia—whose immune systems are already compromised—to let infections go unchecked. If your dentist indicates that you need root canal therapy, please do not delay the procedure. Understand why you need the treatment, discuss your options and decide to either have the tooth treated or have it pulled. Of course, when possible, saving the tooth is always preferable.

18

COSMETIC DENTISTRY

Making a Lasting Impression

If eyes were made for seeing,
then Beauty is its own excuse for being.
—*Ralph Waldo Emerson*

Just because you have fibromyalgia, there is no reason you can't have a beautiful smile; but remember that a beautiful smile is necessarily a healthy smile. A healthy, beautiful smile will not only make an impact on those who look at you, but also will make you feel good about yourself. People remember a beautiful smile, just as an unhealthy smile exposing cracked, stained, decay-ridden teeth, makes a long-lasting impact. This feeling of increased well-being will give you the additional confidence you may need to continue to cope with your disease.

An independent study conducted through the American Academy of Cosmetic Dentistry (ACD) revealed that 97.7 percent of all Americans feel a beautiful smile is an important social asset. This becomes obvious when you think about how far the career of someone like Julia Roberts would go if she had crooked, stained teeth that showed lots of black fillings every time she appeared flashing that big smile on the screen. The American Academy of Cosmetic Dentistry asked two questions in their survey and collected the following responses, listed in descending order of popularity:

1. What is the first thing you notice in a person's smile?
   - How straight their teeth are
   - Whiteness and color
   - Cleanliness of teeth
   - Sincerity of smile
   - Any missing teeth
   - Sparkle of smile
2. What do you think makes a smile unattractive?
   - Discolored, stained teeth
   - Missing teeth
   - Crooked teeth
   - Decayed teeth
   - Gaps and spaces
   - Dirty teeth

Should You Consider Cosmetic Dentistry?

The following are some questions to ask yourself to determine if it's time to find out what your options are for a more beautiful smile.

- Do you hate to smile in photos?
- Do you immediately hold your hand in front of your mouth when you smile or laugh?
- Do you hold your lip a certain way to avoid showing your teeth when you speak to someone?
- Do you feel your teeth are too dark, crooked, misshaped, or chipped?

If your response is "yes" to any of these questions, look in the mirror and smile, noticing what others see when they look at you. If you don't like what you see, you can benefit from cosmetic dentistry. With the many modern techniques available, in just two or three visits to the dentist, it's possible to transform just about any smile into the "Hollywood makeover."

Any or all of the techniques listed below can be utilized to bring this about, based on your needs and situation:

Bleaching or Whitening the Teeth

Although we call it whitening the teeth, no one actually has pure "white" teeth, but various shades of white, cream, ivory, or yellow. Age, genetics, smoking, and certain foods tend to discolor the teeth. There are three types of stains. *Surface stains* are caused by food. Red wine, coffee, tea, cola, and blueberries are some foods that will discolor teeth. Besides food and certain liquids, other agents may stain the teeth. Whether through smoking or smokeless tobacco use, tobacco will certainly stain teeth if you don't remove its residues daily. Certain medications such as tetracycline (an antibiotic) and chlorhexedine gluconate (used for the treatment of gum disease) are also known to stain teeth. These stains can be managed if removed daily with good home oral hygiene and regular professional cleanings. After a visit to your dentist for a cleaning, you may notice your teeth are considerably brighter with removal of these surface stains.

If you clench and grind your teeth (which is common with those living with fibromyalgia and is discussed in Chapter Fifteen), or you frequently chew ice, pencils, fingernails or other hard objects, you can cause tiny, hairline fractures or cracks to your teeth. These cracks can trap stains from food, beverages, or tobacco and make the discoloration more difficult to remove. These types of stain are commonly called *intrinsic stains*, because they essentially become part of the tooth structure. You may not even notice you're causing these tiny cracks until you see a dark line (caused by a stain) running vertically on a front tooth. You could also be born with these types of intrinsic stains due to some trauma or antibiotics use (mostly tetracycline) you or your mother may have experienced before you were born but when your teeth were developing. These stains usually appear as bands of gray and brown or as white spots.

If you received excessive amounts of fluoride as a child, your teeth might be discolored with a chalky look to them. This is known as *fluorosis* and is also an intrinsic stain. Trauma to a tooth can cause nerve damage and make the tooth appear brown. With root canal therapy, if a crown is not placed over a tooth, the tooth will eventually turn a gray shade and may get darker over time.

The third type of stain is due to *plaque and tartar*. If you don't clean your teeth daily and receive routine professional cleanings, plaque and tartar will give your teeth a brown-stained look. Bleaching works well for removing stains if the teeth are uniformly yellow or brown. If teeth are gray or multi-shaded, then the process may not be very successful. Old fillings can give the appearance of discoloration to teeth. Teeth whitening will not help in this situation. Replacing the fillings with the appropriate cosmetic restoration, after whitening the other teeth, may be the treatment of choice.

There are several different methods used to whiten teeth:

1. Over-the-counter teeth-whitening products. These include whitening toothpaste, strips, paint-on products, and gel and tray kits.

   Teeth-Whitening Toothpaste: The number of brands in this category is increasing daily with advertisers claiming that their products whiten your teeth just by brushing. However, if you're expecting whiter teeth with just toothpaste, you may be disappointed. This category mostly uses an abrasive such as silica, calcium carbonate, di-calcium phosphate, and baking soda to remove stains. Other brands may use a mild whitening agent called titanium dioxide. At best, whitening toothpastes temporarily remove superficial stains.

   Whitening Strips: Procter & Gamble, using its *Crest* brand, was the first company to introduce this type of product. The strips use a peroxide-based chemical to whiten teeth. The whitening effect of this product is similar to the tray technique that uses ten percent carbamide peroxide as the bleaching agent. The advantage to these strips is that they are easy to use.

The disadvantage is that they may slide on the teeth and not stay in place, therefore not producing a uniform result. The strips are only placed on the front teeth, and are therefore not helpful for people who want to whiten the back and in-between the teeth.

Paint-on Teeth-Whitening Products: These come in over-night types (Colgate *Simply White Night,* Crest *Night Effects*) and others that are used during the day. In this category, most people seem to agree that the ones that are left on the teeth overnight are more effective.

Gel with Tray Kits: Teeth-whitening became popular when dentists began dispensing kits in the late 1980s. The kits consisted of custom-made mouth trays and syringes containing ten percent carbamide peroxide as the bleaching agent. Since then, infomercials are flooding television and radio almost daily with these products and store shelves display numerous brands. These over-the-counter brands typically cost from $30–$60. If you choose one of these products, carefully follow the manufacturer's instructions for best results. Be prepared: sometimes they work well and sometimes they don't. If you don't achieve desired results, don't continue to use them.

All teeth-whitening gels are similar, whether you purchase them at the drug store or the dental office. However, there are some advantages to purchasing them from your dentist:

◆ Your dentist knows if you are a good candidate for teeth whitening and under supervision, you will have better, safer results.

◆ Some over-the-counter whitening systems are nothing more than whitening toothpaste and may not be effective. These products are not regulated by the F.D.A. because they are considered cosmetic.

◆ The mouth trays made in the dental office are more closely fitted and deliver the bleach uniformly to all the teeth. The trays that have to be boiled and fitted in the over-the-counter kits often do not fit as well.

♦ Some people get obsessed with wanting their teeth "white," and they just never seem white enough. This may lead to overuse and abuse of the whitening agent and cause sensitivity and weakening of the teeth. Although your teeth may have become slightly whiter, you may not notice it since you don't have a true record of their previous color. With a dentist's supervision, this can be avoided. The dentist takes before and after "shades" and even close-up photos of the teeth and can offer other options if this technique fails to produce the desired effect.

2. Teeth whitening procedures that are available from the dentist. Professional brands offer kits for dental offices that include trays that conform more snuggly to your teeth than the boil-and-fit mouth trays available in over-the-counter kits.

Opalescence is one such product that includes the gel in an inner tray package, contained in an outer tray. Both trays are placed in the mouth. The outer tray is removed immediately, and the thin inner tray is gently molded to the teeth. No boiling is required, and the thin, inner tray is not bulky, but pliable, and easily conforms to the teeth. The product can whiten front and back teeth. This type of kit usually costs between eighty-nine and one hundred dollars. The kits that require custom trays require two appointments and are more expensive than the whitening kits that come with trays. To make the custom trays, the dentist or assistant takes molds of your upper and lower teeth. You return in a week or two and take home the kit, which consists of custom trays and whitening gel syringes. You're given instructions on how to use the kit, and the shade of your existing teeth is taken and recorded in your patient chart. This system also takes from a few days to a week to see results. Cost for kits with custom trays vary from about $200 to $500.

In-office whitening. This procedure is done in the dental office and often takes one to two hours. A high intensity light may be used and the dentist or registered dental assistant

(R.D.A.) applies the whitening gel, tooth by tooth. This system works well especially if you have sensitive teeth. A special barrier covers areas that are sensitive so the bleach doesn't touch those areas. This is the most effective way to whiten the teeth. Since the bleach is applied directly to the teeth, the teeth become whiter and it only takes one or two visits at the most, instead of several days. The cost for in-office bleaching is $375 to $1,000. Popular brands include *Britesmile* and *Zoom*.

Tooth-whitening (bleaching) is an excellent way to remove certain types of stains (uniform staining on the teeth, not spots or bands). The best methods are the ones you either obtain from the dentist or have done in the dental office. The advantages to teeth whitening are:

♦ The process is painless with no need of anesthetic.
♦ If you choose the in-office approach you can see results in one appointment—or two at the most.
♦ The technique is fairly inexpensive.
♦ No trimming or alteration of teeth is required.

Are there any disadvantages to teeth-whitening systems, whether purchased over-the-counter or through your dentist? In fact, there are some caveats:

♦ There has been concern about hydrogen peroxide producing "free radicals." Free radicals have been associated with cancer and other degenerative diseases, as well as aging. Studies have shown that enzymes in saliva protect the oral cavity from long-term negative health risks of hydrogen peroxide. It is recommended that smoking be stopped during teeth whitening, because one study found that hydrogen peroxide increased the carcinogenic effects of tobacco. If the product is used within the prescribed time, and under supervision of a dentist, this should not be a problem.
♦ Some at-home over-the-counter whitening products have produced changes in the enamel surface of teeth. The reason

could be that some people leave the product in too long, or that the product has relatively high concentrations of hydrogen peroxide.

♦ Gum sensitivity is common, although mostly temporarily. Studies have shown that peroxide affects the nerve tissue of teeth as it moves from the outer enamel layer to the inner portion. Only very small amounts penetrate the enamel layer, and this accounts for the "zing" that's felt during bleaching. Recession of gums exposes the root surfaces of teeth, which are especially prone to sensitivity. These areas cannot be whitened and should be avoided.

♦ Once teeth are bleached, the process can't be reversed.

♦ Temporary sensitivity to teeth may occur.

♦ The technique simply may not be as effective as you hoped. Normally it should lighten teeth by approximately three to six shades.

♦ Repeated treatments (touch-ups) will be needed in time, depending on the types of stain-producing food, drink, or tobacco you use. Within one and a half to two years, touch-ups may be required.

♦ As for dental fillings, some surface erosion and deterioration of white **composite filling**s have occurred due to the peroxide contact. New amalgam fillings may release mercury during bleaching, and some studies recommend delaying teeth whitening following their initial placement.

Some Final Thoughts on Teeth-whitening.

Most in-office types of whitening use hydrogen peroxide, while most of the take-home types use carbamide peroxide. It takes a higher strength carbamide peroxide to whiten teeth than hydrogen peroxide. The reasons most take-home products use carbamide peroxide is that it acts more slowly before releasing the peroxide. This is why it can be left in the mouth for a few hours at a time. Hydrogen peroxide acts very quickly, yet can be more harmful, and therefore, it's normally delivered in the office within an hour-long appointment. Some take-home products may use hydrogen peroxide instead of carbamide peroxide, but the concentration is usually less than the in-office products. Most take-home types recommended by dentists use ten to fifteen percent carbamide peroxide, while other dentists offer a sixteen to twenty-two percent concentration. The higher strength peroxides should not be left in the mouth for long periods of time.

Ultimately, it's important to ask your dentist which form of whitening is best for you. The results will be more successful when you follow instructions and have realistic expectations.

Some other methods to improve your smile and self-confidence, giving you the inner strength you need to continue to deal with fibromyalgia:

Bonding

+ **Bonding:** If all you see black fillings when you yawn or smile, bonding will help brighten your smile. Bonding (the use of composite or porcelain fillings), is a technique used to replace the mercury silver fillings or used as a filling material on a tooth that has a new cavity on a front or back tooth. Bonding can either be done in the office in one appointment, or made by a laboratory after a mold is taken of the tooth or teeth. If sent to a laboratory to be made, these bonding materials are called "**inlays**" or "**onlay**s" and cost more than the office-placed versions. The laboratory-made white fillings may provide a better fit because the laboratory has a mold of the tooth to work with without the restrictions of saliva, tongue, and the patient's anxiety that the dentist has to manage while placing the filling. The laboratory-made inlays and onlays are usually a stronger material, compared to the composites the dentist uses in the office. Both forms can be made to match the existing teeth, since they come in a variety of shades. The dentist has a shade guide by which to match the color of the bonding to the natural teeth. When these types of fillings were first introduced, they were inferior to the mercury silver fillings. Now, they are just as strong and covered by many insurance plans. Their prices depend on what state, city, community, and even street where the dental office is located. The composite bonded fillings may range in price from $90–$275, while inlays and onlays may cost anywhere from $300 to $1000 or more per tooth, depending on the location of the office.

◆ **Veneers or crowns:** If teeth are misshaped, crooked, or grossly discolored, veneers and/or crowns are the way to make them over. Veneers cover only the front and edge of the tooth and are mostly placed on front and side teeth. Approximately one-eighth of the outer surface of the tooth is trimmed and shaped with a dental drill. A mold is taken and sent to a laboratory. A temporary veneer is placed on the trimmed area and you're sent home with simple care instructions. You return in about two to three weeks for the final veneer to be bonded on the tooth.

With a crown, approximately two millimeters of tooth enamel is removed from the entire tooth. Otherwise, the preparation of a crown follows the same procedure as for a veneer. Interestingly, one indication for a crown could be over-exposure to high levels of chlorine in swimming pools. In a recent issue of the *American Journal of Dentistry*, it was reported that pool water sometimes has levels of chlorine high enough to stain and wear enamel.

◆ **Implants:** The implant is an anchor inserted in the jaw, around which a natural looking tooth is placed. Implants are used for either replacing a missing tooth or for holding dentures in place securely. To anchor dentures, implants are surgically placed in the jaw. Attachments are than installed in the dentures so that when the denture is put in the mouth, the two components snap into place, providing a stable fit.

If you have a missing tooth, and the adjacent teeth are

healthy, without any existing fillings or crowns, then an implant is a good choice. The alternative would require shaping and reducing the size of adjacent teeth to place a permanent bridge that would include a replacement for the missing tooth. With the implant, the adjacent teeth are not affected. However, you have to have strong, healthy bone and gums to be a good candidate for an implant. Your dentist can determine if that is the case.

♦ **Orthodontics:** Teeth can be straightened with braces or the latest technique using mouth trays called Invisalign. Orthodontics may take two to four years to achieve the desired results. Excellent periodontal (supporting structures of the teeth) health is crucial for adult orthodontic treatment, because movement of teeth may cause them to loosen if the gums and bone are not healthy.

♦ **Gum surgery:** This is another method that may achieve cosmetic results. Some people have a "gummy smile," in which all you see is gums when they smile. Gum grafting may be necessary if a person has long teeth, in which the gums have receded.

♦ **Dentures:** Many people have to wear full or **partial dentures**. Most feel they have to live with unattractive teeth. With modern dentistry, partial dentures can be made so that no one will be able to tell dentures from real teeth. Old-fashioned dentures had wire or metal clasps to hold them in place. The modern partial denture has gum colored clasps that blend in. Full dentures can be made with teeth that are very cosmetically natural looking and strong. Implants and other attachments, including holding on to some natural roots of the person's teeth, can also be used to give extra stability to dentures. In this way, the person can feel secure in chewing, without worries that the denture will slip out of the mouth.

I started this chapter by stating that a beautiful smile starts with a healthy smile. Even if you spend thousands of dollars on cosmetic dentistry, but you have bad breath due to gum disease, smoke cigarettes and neglect other needed dental care, then your money was wasted. Learn how to practice proper home oral hygiene, eat a balanced diet and make regular dental visits for check-ups and cleanings. Take care of the foundation of the teeth and then consider cosmetic dentistry as icing on the cake.

Of course, beauty is in the eye of the beholder. Next time you smile at yourself in the mirror, and decide you need a smile over-haul, make an appointment with your dentist and discuss your options. You'll be surprised at the change dental techniques can make in how you feel about yourself and the world around you. On the other side of the coin, it's not healthy to get too obsessed with looks. Be realistic with your dentist in setting your goals and expectations for improving your smile.

19

ALTERNATIVE DENTISTRY

Looking for a Cure

M any people seek "alternative" means of care for their health conditions. Authors of such alternative methods write books, become gurus, and often grow very wealthy as they make their appearances on infomercials and the talk show circuit. True or not, their promises are appealing: it's not easy, for example, to resist a supplement that is claimed to help you lose your undesired weight and increase your sex drive at the same time. Since there is no cure for fibromyalgia, many wonder if they should explore alternative methods for help and relief of symptoms.

Alternative dentists also make appealing promises and claims. Some allege that removing mercury fillings will cure any disease or lessen the severity of such conditions as chronic fatigue and fibromyalgia. Some say that pulling teeth that have root canals will cure cancer and symptoms related to fibromyalgia. There is no evidence to support any of these claims.

In general, alternative dentistry runs counter to traditional dental treatment methods and recommends herbs, homeopathic remedies, and other means to supplement or provide treatment.

Some methods recommended by alternative dentists are dangerous and completely useless, while others can provide helpful
adjuncts to traditional methods of treatment.

Before getting excited about their promises of cure for
fibromyalgia and spending money on alternative methods for dental treatment, do your research. This chapter will help you understand how dentists can best incorporate useful alternative methods
within traditional dental treatment. Some alternative methods
such as acupuncture may help with relief of your TMJ pain. Foot
reflexology provided at some dental offices can help you relax during treatment, while other alternative modalities may help improve
healing after surgery. These and other forms of alternative dental
treatments will be presented to help you understand what is available and how they can help you with your fibromyalgia.

Acupuncture

In dentistry, acupuncture has been evaluated for use in pain
management, as an alternative to dental anesthetics, as a method
to help with the gagging reflex, to overcome phobias and anxiety,
and to stimulate salivation. The most successful use has been in
managing pain in people suffering from facial pain and temporomandibular joint disorder (TMJ) that affects the jaw joint and
often causes facial pain, headaches, and ringing in the ears,
among other symptoms. This disorder is common among people
living with fibromyalgia. Therefore if you have fibromyalgia, you
might consider acupuncture as an adjunct to traditional treatment
modes.

The traditional form of treatment of TMJ is a multidisciplinary
approach including fabrication of an "occlusal splint" or mouthguard made by the dentist, physical therapy, chiropractic adjustments, or medical specialty care such as ENT (otolaryngology) for
diagnosis and treatment of other symptoms associated with TMJ.
Several studies suggest that acupuncture can be effective in

reducing the pain associated with TMJ in only a few treatments. The regimen studied consisted of at least six treatments given weekly, with needles placed in specific points related to TMJ.

Acupuncture seems to lessen pain by affecting neurotransmitters. We experience pain when certain specific signals are transmitted to pain cells in the brain. Acupuncture needles appear to activate small nerve fibers in muscle, which send impulses to the spinal cord and then activate the midbrain. As a needle is placed in an acupuncture point, a small inflammatory process occurs which releases neurotransmitters such as bradykinin, histamine, and others. A chain reaction results, by which "layer IV neurons" release a substance called "enkephaline." This substance inhibits incoming painful sensations by attaching to pain nerves and blocking activation of the pain-perceiving cells in the medulla (the lowermost part of the brain).

Using acupuncture instead of local anesthetic to dampen sensation seems to be effective for minor dental visits only, such as cleanings. For more extensive treatment, unless you were brought up with the use of acupuncture or have low pain tolerance, traditional local anesthetic works better. An advantage to local anesthetic is that it takes only seconds to minutes to achieve the desired effect, while acupuncture may take twenty to thirty minutes. More studies are needed to furnish data on how successful neural therapy (see below) and traditional acupressure are for managing pain during dental treatment. However, these techniques have been shown to be helpful following dental treatment, especially for people who can't tolerate traditional pain medications.

Most alternative practitioners believe conventional medicine can be harmful to your health, while the "natural" alternative techniques are totally safe. There have been reports, however, of adverse effects following acupuncture treatment. These include pneumothorax (collection of air or gas in the space surrounding the lungs), endocarditis (infection involving the heart), and hepatitis. These effects could be due to an inexperienced acupuncturist or one who did not apply prudent sterilization methods in treating patients. In general, acupuncture is safe in the hands of a trained and qualified practitioner.

Many alternative dentists use neural therapy. A German physician, Reinhold Voll, originally formulated this method of diagnosis and treatment in the 1950s. He observed that each tooth in the mouth is somehow connected to and affects a certain pathway of acupuncture energy (called a *meridian*). If a bodily organ is not functioning properly, the tooth related to that organ via a meridian may be painful. For example, if a person has kidney or bladder problems, probing a lower or upper front tooth may cause tenderness. Dr. David J. Schuch recently presented information about this concept at the 49th Annual Meeting of the Academy of General Dentistry in New York.

In one instance, a patient of Dr. Schuch had a fifteen-year history of stomach ulcers and was on medication to reduce gastric acid. After removal of an infected lower premolar (which, this theory goes, is linked to the stomach) the ulcers and symptoms disappeared. For years, another patient of Dr. Schuch suffered from chronic internal pain near his navel. Specialists were unable to diagnose the problem. After removing two infected lower left molars (which are related to the small intestine), his lower abdominal pain disappeared. Of course, these are only two instances that claim support for this theory. More thorough research and standardized tests are required to evaluate this relationship.

Since the teeth were infected, it is possible that removing them helped Dr. Schuch's patient feel better. However, be suspicious if a holistic dentist tells you that your fibromyalgia symptoms will improve by pulling teeth that tested negative on his "machine." Many of these "machines" used by holistic dentists to determine disease in teeth as related to other organs do not have FDA approval.

Other uses of needle-less acupuncture in dentistry are the stimulation of the point "Nei Guan" to help control the gagging reflex during dental treatment. Another acupuncture point called "Hoku" (also called "Rokou," "HeGu") is helpful for dental pain and can be stimulated by the patient. This is located between the

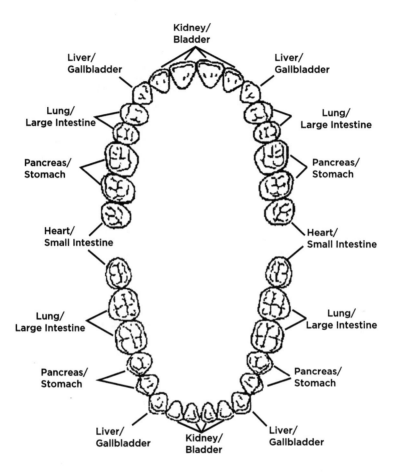

Figure 5 Acupuncture Points Related to Dentition (Courtesy of The Academy of General Dentistry)

thumb and index finger, and can be stimulated to decrease pain during dental treatment.

Dr. Paul Nogier first introduced ear acupuncture, called auricular therapy. He indicated that the outer ear could be viewed as an inverted fetus, with the head at the bottom of the ear, the feet at the top, and the body in the middle. The jaw and teeth are located in the middle of the lobe can be stimulated for conditions related to those areas.

Foot Reflexology

Reflexology uses massage on various points and regions on the feet to provide relief for stress and tension. In dentistry, many offices that are using a "spa" approach to relax patients offer foot reflexology for relief of anxiety before and during treatment. Foot reflexology is a wonderful way to reduce stress and promote relaxation. Claims that stimulating certain points on the foot will cure disease are still under investigation.

One theory of how foot reflexology reduces stress is through the nervous system. As the foot is massaged, local "peripheral" nerves send signals to the central nervous system that stimulates various parts of the brain. The brain makes adjustments on levels of oxygen and blood supply that effect overall physical tone and tension of the body.

Various methods and tools are used for foot reflexology. The area can be massaged by hand or products such as wooden wands or motorized foot rests used.

Herbs and Supplements

For management of fibromyalgia symptoms, you may be taking several medications. This is why it is very important not to take any herbs without discussion with your physician. Herbs can be powerful sources of drugs and should not be taken lightly, especially if you are taking medications. Many people think just because herbs are natural they are safe. If the bottle says to take one, they may think taking three or four may be even better. What they don't understand is that you can just as easily overdose with herbal supplements as you can with traditional drugs. Traditional drugs are regulated and tested, while many herbal supplements are not regulated and there is no well-established standard for dosage and effects.

Most drugs were originally derived from herbs, but once a chemical ingredient within the herb is found to produce a therapeutic effect, it can usually be manufactured synthetically. Natural or synthetic, the active ingredient is largely the same and can cause adverse effects. It is important not to take supplements based on an article you've read, but upon recommendation of your physician.

Below is a list of some common herbs and supplements used in alternative dentistry:

- *Aloe vera*: is applied to cold cores for relief of symptoms. A study published in *General Dentistry*, the journal of the Academy of General Dentistry indicated that aloe vera may helpful heal of cold sores inside and outside of the mouth. According to J. Michael Adame, DDS, **FAGD**, former pharmacist and spokesperson for the Academy of General Dentistry, "In addition to its anti-viral and anti-inflammatory properties, aloe vera provides benefits to the skin, such as amino acids, B_1, B_2, B_6, and C vitamins." Dr. Adame recommends that cold sore sufferers apply aloe vera balm three times per day until the **lesion** has dried. "It will combat the sore and enhance healing," he said.
- *Anise* has anti-inflammatory properties. It could help relieve inflammation associated with gum disease, if used as a mouth rinse.
- *Chamomile* relieves pain and anxiety prior to dental treatment.
- *Cloves*: oil of cloves has been used to ease tooth pain.
- *Vitamin C*: deficiency of this vitamin could cause bleeding gums.
- *Coenzyme Q10*: some studies indicate this may be beneficial for treatment of gum disease.

Inform your dentist if you are taking any herbs. This is important because some herbs may have negative effects. For example,

St. John's Wort and other herbs that are meant to help you relax may lead to excess sedation when taken with a prescription drug. Gingko may cause bleeding of the gums because it has an effect on platelets and the clotting mechanism.

Homeopathy

Homeopathy uses plants, minerals, or animals in very small doses as remedies. Its premise is that if too much of a substance (such as arsenic) brings about harmful symptoms, that same substance in very small amounts will remove the symptoms. This principle of homeopathy is known as the "law of similars" and bears some resemblance to the vaccines used for immunizations in traditional medicine. For dosages and recommended use of homeopathic products, read the instructions on the package. Homeopathic practitioners claim that mint and coffee may undermine the effectiveness of homeopathic remedies. You should understand that homeopathy is an experimental field and that no scientific studies have established its validity.

Common homeopathic remedies used by alternative dentists include:

- Aconite: for help with fear and anxiety of dental treatment.
- Arnica (mountain daisy): used for traumatic injury and pain associated with it. Used frequently for TMJ pain.
- Belladonna (deadly nightshade): to treat swelling and fever accompanying an abscess.
- Borax: to treat dry mouth, canker sores.
- Capsicum: to treat oral herpes.
- Chamomile: for help with tooth pain brought on by hot or warm foods or drinks.
- Hyperacid (St. John's Wort): for pain involving the nerves, following root canal therapy or tooth extraction.
- Ipecacuanha (ipecac): for bleeding.

- Plantago (plantain): for help with toothache that radiates pain to ear.
- Silicea: For gums that are sensitive to cold.
- Xerophyllum: for TMJ symptoms.

As a caution: If you choose to explore the use of herbs and homeopathic remedies, consult with a physician who has been trained in the field. Inform your dentist if you are taking any herbs or homeopathic remedies.

Appendix

Dental Problem Guide

If you are living with fibromyalgia, the last thing you need is to have a dental emergency and not know what to do. Dental emergencies don't often occur in the United States because most people have quick access to a dentist. However, there are times, whether on a weekend or on holidays, when emergencies occur and it's just not possible to get in touch with your dentist. This guide will help you stay calm during those times and be able to take appropriate action. You'll also learn what a particular type of dental pain means; for example, toothache can be sharp and quick, dull and intermittent or a constant aching. These all signal a different problem with a tooth. Refer to Chapter 15 on finding a dentist so that if an emergency does occur, you won't have to deal with the burden of finding a dentist at such a time.

The topics are divided into three sections. Section one gives guidance for tooth pain. The type of pain you're feeling could be important information to help you decide what the cause is and how quickly you should get to the dentist. The second part gives information on what to do if there are problems with the jaw. The last section helps with problems that involve dentures, bridges, or crowns. Of course, you must seek professional help as soon as possible for all dental conditions—the earlier the better, because prolonging a minor condition without treatment can advance to major costly problems.

Tooth Pain Interpretation

All teeth are composed of three layers. The outer layer is called **enamel**, is very hard and covers and protects the crown of the tooth, which is the portion that is visible above the gums. The layer directly beneath enamel is called **dentin**. Dentin is softer than enamel and has a slightly yellow shade. If dentin is exposed to air from wear or fracture of enamel, you may feel sensitivity. Below dentin is the **pulp**, which contains the blood supply that carries nutrients to the tooth, and the nerves (that will let you know loudly and clearly if there is a problem with the tooth).

Dental pain can be misleading. Pain in an upper molar may come from a sinus infection, while a new filling or crown that needs the bite adjusted could cause pain radiating to the ear area. Pain as a reaction to hot, cold and sweets could mean you need a filling or that there is an infection in the tooth and root canal therapy is needed. This is why the dentist requires X-rays of teeth to diagnose properly. X-rays, along with the type of pain you've been experiencing, and an examination of the area all help determine appropriate treatment.

The source of most common toothaches is tooth decay. The process usually starts with plaque, that clear film that covers all the teeth and if not removed disguises colonies of bacteria causing endless trouble in the mouth. Bacteria produce acid during fermentation of carbohydrates and other foods such as meats, bread or sugar, and demineralize tooth structure, the process that we call decay. If the decay is not cleaned out and the area restored by a filling material, destruction spreads to deeper levels until the nerve of the tooth is reached in the pulp chamber. Pain may be felt at any stage once demineralization starts, but it increases as it gets closer to the nerve. Once it reaches the nerve, irreversible damage occurs and root canal therapy will be necessary. The only other option will be to extract (pull) the tooth. If appropriate treatment occurs in a timely manner, root canal therapy or extraction will be avoided.

TOOTH PAIN AND WHAT IT COULD MEAN

Symptom	Possible Cause	What the dentist may do
Sensitivity to cold foods that only lasts momentarily and subsides and does not recur.	This may not be a problem at all but due to a tooth being exposed to cold food or drink, or a momentary trauma such as biting on hard food.	
Sensitivity to cold, hot, or sweet foods that lasts momentarily but returns every time you eat cold, hot, or sweet foods without having had recent dental work.	May be a sign of a loose filling, or a slight crack in the tooth or filling. Also may be due to gum recession that has exposed the root surface. This area is susceptible to sensitivity because it is softer than enamel.	Avoid eating very hot or cold foods or liquids on that side and see your dentist for an evaluation. You will either need a filling or a crown. Eventually, you may also need root canal therapy depending on proximity of problem to the pulp. Note if you are brushing too hard or clenching and grinding your teeth, which will cause gum recession and expose the root surface. In this case you may need a mouth guard.
Toothache after eating popcorn or other foods that you think may have gotten lodged under the gums.	Not cleaning out food lodged under the gums is a contributing factor to gum disease, pain, and inflammation.	Rinse your mouth with warm water and gently floss between the teeth, extending the floss under the gums. Never use a sharp object to try to check under the gums. If the pain and discomfort continue, see your dentist to help clean it out. **Caution:** Never put aspirin or other painkillers directly on the gums or it may cause a chemical burn.

Pain with hot, cold or sweets, comes and goes on its own.	Known as *reversible pulpitis,* this involves inflammation of the pulp tissue.	See your dentist. You may require a filling.
Pain is very severe in reaction to hot, cold or sweets and does not go away.	Irreversible pulp inflammation, this is also inflammation of the pulp tissue, but more advanced because it was not treated during initial reversible stage.	See your dentist; you will need either a root canal or to get the tooth pulled.
Pain on chewing following dental treatment.	It is not unusual to have some discomfort after recent dental treatment. However, this may indicate you need a bite adjustment.	Don't chew on that side and don't clench your teeth on that side until you see your dentist. A simple bite adjustment should relieve the pain.
Pain on chewing without recent dental work, cold sensitivity only.	Could be sign of fracture/crack in filling or tooth.	Avoid that side and see your dentist as soon as possible. You may need a filling or a crown restoration.
Pain on chewing, hot sensitivity that lingers.	Inflamed pulp tissue will react painfully to hot foods, liquids, or chewing. There may be a fracture or decay in the tooth.	See your dentist as soon as possible. You will probably require root canal therapy.
Constant, severe pain accompanied by swelling from hot and cold.	Irreversible pulp inflammation.	The affected tooth may require root canal therapy or extraction. If there is swelling, you will need antibiotics. Contact a dentist as soon as possible or go to an emergency room at the closest hospital and get some antibiotics until you can see a dentist.
Tenderness on tapping a tooth after root canal therapy.	Gum inflammation of the "periodontal" attachments that connect the gums to the tooth.	See your dentist for evaluation. You may only require a bite adjustment or other minor treatment.

Constant, severe pain to hot and cold, or chewing with swelling.	Irreversible pulp inflammation.	Tooth may likely require root canal therapy extraction. If there is swelling, you will need antibiotics. Contact a dentist as soon as possible or go to an emergency room at the closest hospital and get some antibiotics until you can see a dentist.
Gum boil (swelling) and pain surrounding a tooth.	Infection in the gums or tooth abscess.	See your dentist for evaluation and treatment for either a root canal or to extract (pull) a tooth. You'll need antibiotic therapy as well.
Swelling that looks like it's spreading to the neck or cheeks, accompanied by severe pain.	Known as *cellulitis,* this infection may have started with a tooth or gum area, but is now spreading. The lymph glands become tender and there is fever.	Your dentist will prescribe antibiotics, and you'll need either root canal therapy or extraction of a tooth. You will probably need to have the infection drained. Serious complications may occur if the infection spreads to the head and neck, compromising the airway and even causing further complications involving the central nervous system. Hospitalization may be needed.
Tooth cracks (fracture).	Broken tooth.	You'll need a filling, crown, root canal therapy, or to have the tooth removed, depending on extent of fracture. Avoid the area and see your dentist ASAP.
Loose tooth.	Either from gum disease or trauma.	Gum treatment; splinting of the tooth to other teeth or with a fixed or removable appliance; possible root canal therapy.
Swelling and pain behind the very last tooth in the lower jaw.	Commonly called "pericoronitis", this problem is usually related to an unerupted or partially erupted tooth (usually a wisdom tooth).	Rinse with warm salt water (one cup warm water to one tsp. salt) as often as needed for relief. See your dentist for evaluation and treatment including antibiotics, if infection is present; extraction; or irrigation under the gums in the area. Lymph glands may be swollen and you may not be able to open your mouth fully (trismus).

Knocked out tooth.	This is common with kids who are active in sports. To prevent these types of accidents, a sports guard is recommended.	Hold the tooth by the crown and gently rinse with water. DO NOT SCRUB or you will destroy important tissue that is needed to reattach the tooth in the socket. If possible place the tooth back in the socket and immediately go to the dentist. If this is not possible, place the tooth either under the tongue or in a container with milk so it doesn't dry and get to the dentist ASAP. The sooner the dentist can replant the tooth in the socket (ideally within half an hour), the better the chances of saving the tooth. This applies to permanent teeth only. Baby (primary) teeth are not replanted.
Tooth has been pushed into the gum from trauma (intrusion), where it's nearly invisible.	Common in children who are active and not using a sports guard to protect the teeth.	The tooth may erupt on its own, or may have to be guided surgically or orthodontically.

Acceptable mediums in which to store a tooth that has fallen out

- Milk (fat content does not matter)
- Cold water
- Saline
- In your mouth, under the tongue

Problems with the Jaw

Because the jaw is associated with to the head and neck, problems with the jaw may show signs and symptoms in the neck, head, and most structures of the face including the eyes, ears, and sinuses. Symptoms can become very intense and, unfortunately, can also be very misleading. Although the cause could be the jaw radiating pain to the sides of the head, causing pressure with pain behind the eyes, and ringing in the ears, it is easy to misdiagnose and not even consider the jaw as a possible cause of any of these symptoms. Below is a chart of possible problems associated with jaw:

JAW PROBLEMS, CAUSES AND SOLUTIONS

Symptom	Possible Cause	What the dentist may do
All your teeth ache or just those on one side. You can't pinpoint any one tooth.	You may be grinding or clenching the teeth. If the symptoms disappear and do not return, it was a one-time situation from trauma or stress.	Consciously keep your teeth apart and eat soft foods for a few days until the aching is not felt. In the meantime, see your dentist if this occurs often, for TMJ evaluation.
Noises in the ears, pain on opening and/or closing the mouth or while chewing.	Possible TMJ.	Consciously keep your teeth apart and eat soft foods. See your dentist for TMJ evaluation.
Sudden, shock-like, stabbing pain on one side of the jaw or cheek. May last for several seconds and come and go throughout the day, persisting for days, weeks.	Trigenimal neuralgia ("tic douloureux") is a condition that affects the fifth cranial nerve which one of the largest nerves of the head.	Anti-convulsants and pain medication may be prescribed; surgery may be necessary.
Severe trauma to the jaw with accompanying pain.	Possible fracture to the jaw.	To control swelling, apply cold compress. Go to a hospital emergency room or dentist. Hold the jaw immobile as much as possible until you reach help.

Emergencies Involving Crowns, Bridges, or Dentures

Crowns and permanent bridges should last anywhere from five to fifteen years. Chewing on sticky foods, such as taffy, may loosen a crown or bridge. Removable dentures may have their own emergencies, such as a tooth falling out or fractures.

PROBLEMS WITH CROWNS, BRIDGES, AND DENTURES

Symptom	Possible Cause	What the dentist may do
Temporary or permanent crown or bridge comes off.	If a permanent crown, chewing sticky foods is one cause or there may be underlying decay, loosening the crown. It's not uncommon for temporary crowns to come off, because temporary cements are used.	Purchase denture adhesive (salicylate free if on guaifenesin protocol) from a drugstore. Rinse the crown clean of food debris and dab a small amount of adhesive into the crown; place back on tooth until you can see your dentist. You may need a new crown, or your dentist may re-cement the old one after disinfecting and cleaning it.
Chipped or broken denture.	Old dentures may fracture with wear, or from dropping or other accident.	Do not place a chipped or broken denture in your mouth, especially if it has sharp edges. Leave it out of your mouth until you see your dentist. If you cannot see a dentist for a few days, you can purchase a temporary repair kit from many drugstores.
Tooth falls out of a removable denture.	Biting on a hard food can loosen a tooth, or, if the denture is old, teeth may occasionally break off.	Keep the tooth and take it to the dentist. This may save you money if the dentist can place the same tooth back on the denture. Otherwise, a new tooth will be created to replace the lost or broken one.

With the first sign of any symptoms, it's always safer to seek professional help, if nothing else, just for peace of mind. If any symptom comes and goes, don't wait for it to get worse. If you're going to be leaving on any extended vacations or other trips, get a check-up before leaving. Health care in foreign countries may be costly and not up to American standards. I don't recommend leaving on a trip while in the middle of dental treatment. If it cannot be helped, take along the items listed below so you'll be prepared if the need arises.

Emergency Dental Kit for Home or Travel

- A container to hold the needed items.
- Small mirror (if possible, a mouth mirror made for dental purposes available at most drugstores).
- Small flashlight.
- Temporary filling available at drugstores, in case a filling falls out. (A note of caution: If there is an infection in the tooth, and a filling has fallen out, closing the opening with a temporary filling may cause pressure to build up, with resulting intense pain.)
- Aspirin.
- Cotton swabs.
- Small bottles of alcohol-free antiseptic mouthwash.
- Gauze bandages.
- Temporary dental cement, available at drugstores, to repair crowns or bridges that fall out (if you have crowns or bridges in your mouth).
- Temporary denture repair kit (if you have a full or partial denture).
- If you have children who are active with sports, take a container with milk in case a tooth is knocked out. You can place the tooth in the container and get it and the child to the dentist as soon as possible. However, to prevent teeth from falling out, use a sports guard.

Glossary

ABRASION. Wear of tooth structure due to mechanical means such as brushing too hard.

ABSCESS. A pocket that forms filled with pus, and may be an acute or chronic localized inflammation often with swelling, associated with a tooth, teeth, or the gums. As pressure builds up, can be painful.

ABUTMENT, IMPLANT. Part of the implant that is anchored to the jawbone to which the crown (part that looks like a tooth) is attached.

ABUTMENT, TOOTH. An anchor tooth used to support a false tooth replacing a missing tooth.

ACID ETCHING. Phosphoric acid solution used to prepare the enamel surface of a tooth for retention before bonding.

ACUPUNCTURE. A technique, which originated in China, for curing disease, relieving pain, or bringing about partial anesthesia by inserting needles into the body at specific points.

ADA. American Dental Association located in Chicago, IL.

AIR ABRASION. A dental tool that utilizes a "sand-blasting" type of technique to remove small cavities without anesthetic.

ALGINATE. An impression material used to make molds of the teeth and mouth for study models and fabrication of prosthetics such as dentures.

ALPHA ACTIVITY. EEG oscillations with a frequency of 8–13 Hz in adults; indicative of the awake state; present in most, but not all, normal individuals; most consistent and predominant during relaxed wakefulness.

ALVEOLAR BONE. The part of the jawbone that supports the teeth.

ALVEOLOPLASTY. Reshaping and recontouring the jawbone in preparation for a prosthesis such as a denture.

AMALGAM. A material used to fill teeth, consisting of a mixture of mercury with silver, copper, tin, and other materials.

ANAEROBIC BACTERIA. Bacteria that do not need oxygen to grow. The "harmful" bacteria that cause gum disease.

ANALGESIA. Loss of pain. Usually refers to medications or drugs to help alleviate pain.

ANESTHETIC.

Local Anesthetic. Loss of sensation in one local area due to injection of a nerve blocking solution, usually used to "numb" one tooth. Cocaine was the first to be used in the 1860s in Germany. The first synthetic local anesthetic was Novocain (which is no longer used). Lidocaine (Xylocaine) was introduced in the 1940s. Several others were developed producing different effects: mepivocaine, bupivocaine, etidocaine, prilocaine. Some are short-acting, while others are long-acting and don't wear off as quickly. A vasoconstrictor in the form of epinephrine is often added to slow the rate of absorption by the bloodstream, making the anesthetic longer acting. A side effect of epinephrine in anesthetic may be a feeling of "rush" with rapid heart beat and the jitters. If this bothers you and occurs often, you can ask your dentist to use an anesthetic that does not have epinephrine in it. Amount used depends on age, weight, and health. Allergies to local anesthetics are very rare.

Block Anesthetic. Local anesthetic delivered to anesthetize a nerve trunk, often used to treat several teeth next to each other at once. In mandibular block injection, half the jaw, tongue, and teeth on that side will be numb.

Intravenous Sedation (IV Sedation). Intravenous conscious sedation is used on people that have mild to moderate anxiety or fear about the dental treatment. Drugs are administered intravenously and sometimes nitrous oxide through inhalation, to help relax the patient. The person has little memory of the appointment or the treatment received.

General Anesthesia. With this technique, the person becomes totally unconscious and asleep. This is recommended for patients who have severe dental phobias. Intravenous and/or inhalation agents are used.

ANTERIOR TEETH. Front teeth consisting of six teeth on the maxilla (top jaw) and six teeth on the mandible (lower jaw).

ANTIBIOTIC. Medication used to treat infection.

ANTICOAGULANTS. Drugs which prevents or slows down the process of blood forming a clot.

ANTIOXIDANTS. Substances that protects other chemicals of the body from damaging oxidation reactions by reacting with free radicals and other reactive oxygen species within the body, hence hindering the process of oxidation.

A.N.U.G. Acute Necrotizing Ulcerative Gingivitis. Severe and painful form of acute gum infection, commonly called "trench mouth." Must be treated with antibiotics and gum treatments.

APEX. The very end of the root tip of a tooth, through which the blood vessels and nerves pass.

APEXIFICATION. A special type of root canal treatment for developing permanent teeth that allows the root of the tooth to continue developing and forming although the nerve has been injured. The cause of injury is usually due to trauma. Medication is placed in the root canal and may have to be replaced as needed for healing. The process may take from six to twenty-four months to achieve complete development of the root.

APICOECTOMY. When conventional root canals fail, "Apico" consists of surgically amputating the end of the root tip and sealing it with a dental material.

APTHOUS ULCER (see canker sore).

ARGININE. A bitter tasting amino acid found in proteins and necessary for nutrition.

ARTHROPLASTY. Surgical reconstruction or replacement of a malformed or degenerated joint.

ATTRITION. Gradual wear of the teeth; may be due to grinding the teeth.

AUTOANTIBODIES. Antibodies that react with self-antigens (autoantigens) of the organism that produced them.

AUTOCLAVE. A tank-like device for heating substances above their boiling point; used to manufacture chemicals or sterilize surgical instruments.

AUTOGENIC RELAXATION. Similar in many aspects to meditation and self-hypnosis, a technique that helps the patient to activate the body's internal capabilities for healing. It consists of a series of simple exercises that join the mind and body through deep relaxation.

AUTOIMMUNE DISORDER. A disease that results when the immune system attacks the body's own tissues, as in rheumatoid arthritis.

AUTOIMMUNE RESPONSE. This is a reaction of the immune system whereby it attacks normal body issue and confuses it for an "intruder" or harmful tissue.

BENIGN. Diseased tissue that is not recurrent or progressive; not malignant (not spreading to surrounding areas).

BICUSPID (Pre-molar). Two teeth with two points (cusps) situated between the **canine**s and molars on either side of top and bottom jaw. They are located directly in front of the molars.

BILATERAL. Pertaining to both sides.

BIOFEEDBACK. Behavior training program that teaches a person how to control certain autonomic reactions such as heart rate, blood pressure, skin temperature, and muscular tension.

BIOPSY. Removal of a small piece of tissue for laboratory evaluation.

BITEWINGS. Dental radiographs (X-rays) taken with the teeth held together. These show several teeth at once, and allow the dentist to see cavities that have developed between the teeth. Only show the upper 1/3 of the roots.

BLEACHING. Eliminating stains or discolorations by means of an oxidizing agent to improve esthetics. Can be done at home or in the dental office.

BONDING. A technique to place a white filling (plastic or porcelain) in a tooth or to correct cosmetically challenged teeth in order to close gaps, change shades, or straighten crooked teeth.

BONE GRAFT. The placement of artificial, synthetic, or natural bone into areas of the jaw, around teeth, or implants.

BRIDGE (Cantiliver). A fixed bridge that has only one end anchored or supported by a tooth or teeth. The supporting teeth must be very strong or this type of bridge will fail.

BRIDGE (Fixed). A dental appliance that uses teeth on either side of a space as anchors to replace a missing tooth or teeth. Can be made to span one or several teeth. Once this is cemented in place, it cannot be taken out, unless the dentist removes it. Also called "Fixed Bridge."

BRIDGE (Maryland). A type of fixed bridge that requires little tooth removal or preparation, by which thin metal "wings" are acid-etched to the back of abutment teeth anchoring the false tooth in place.

BRIDGE (Removable). A removable appliance used to replace missing teeth. Uses metal or acrylic clasps or implants to anchor it in place. Must be removed and cleaned daily.

BRUXISM. Abnormal grinding of the teeth.

BURNING MOUTH SYNDROME (BMS). A burning pain in the

tongue or other oral mucous membranes associated with normal signs and laboratory findings.

CALCIUM FLUORIDE (CAF2). Also known as fluorite or fluorspar, a naturally occurring mineral and the type found in natural fluoridated water.

CALCULUS. The dental or scientific name given to tartar, which is the calcified deposit of mineralized plaque that attaches to all tooth surfaces. Once it forms, cannot be removed by brushing, but only by professional cleaning using special instruments.

CANAL. A narrow chamber or channel located within each root of the tooth through which flow the blood vessels and nerve to each tooth.

CANDIDA (ORAL). A yeast infection of the mucous membranes of the mouth and tongue.

CANINE (cuspid, or eyetooth). Also known as cuspids, these teeth are situated at the corners of the mouth and are more pointed than other front teeth.

CANKER SORE. Small painful, irritating ulcer that forms in the mouth. Canker sores can be caused by irritants in toothpaste, trauma, stress, or nutritional deficiencies. Also called "recurrent aphthous ulcers."

CAPSAICIN. Colorless pungent crystalline compound derived from capsicum; source of the hotness of hot peppers of the genus Capsicum such as chili and cayenne and jalapeno.

CARIES. Tooth decay.

CAVITY. Any decayed area of a tooth.

CELLULITE. Site of acute inflammation of the connective tissue of the skin, caused by infection with staphylococcus, streptococcus, or other bacteria.

CEMENT. A material used to hold restorations in a tooth.

CEMENT BASE. Material used under a filling as a liner, as deemed necessary by the dentist.

CEMENTUM. The connective tissue covering the root surface of teeth. It is softer than enamel (outer surface of crown of teeth) and when exposed due to receded gums, will cause sensitivity.

CHRONIC FATIGUE SYNDROME. Severe disabling fatigue which lasts at least six months, made worse by minimal physical or mental exertion, and for which there is no adequate medical explanation.

CHRONIC OBSTRUCTIVE PULMONARY DISEASE (COPD). A group of lung diseases involving limited airflow and varying degrees of air sac enlargement, airway inflammation, and lung tissue destruction. Emphysema and chronic bronchitis are the most common forms of COPD.

CLEFT PALATE (hare lip). Congenital deformity that causes incomplete fusion of the hard and soft palate (roof of the mouth). This results in abnormal formation of the nose and lip.

CLENCHING. Abnormal habit of consciously or unconsciously holding the teeth together with excessive force.

COENZYME Q10. A substance that functions as a vitamin and is present inside the cell. Its primary function is an antioxidant which stablizes the membrane activity and prevents depletion of metabolites necessary for the resynthesis of adenosine triphosphate (ATP). The reduced form of the CoQ10 inhibits lipid peroxidation and protects against oxidative stress.

COLD SORE (fever blisters). Herpes Simplex blisters occur mostly on the lips and on the gum area near the teeth. Can reappear without warning. Over-the-counter medication helps with discomfort and healing can be enhanced by some prescription drugs.

COMPOSITE FILLING. A tooth-colored filling material made from a variety of glass particles such as resin and quartz, and used to restore decay in teeth. It is usually hardened by a high intensity light source held over the tooth for ten to sixty seconds after each application.

CRACKED TOOTH SYNDROME. A tooth that has a vertical fracture, seen by the naked eye or not, that is characterized by pain on pressure and cold; may not be evident on X-ray.

C-REACTIVE PROTEIN (CRP). A plasma protein which increases during inflammation. As a blood test, CRP is not specific. A high result serves as a general indication of acute inflammation. Doctors can utilize the CRP test to assess the effectiveness of a specific arthritis treatment and monitor periods of disease flareup.

CREPITATION OR CREPITUS. Sound heard when bone grinds against bone in the jaw joint. This is a result of damaged "disc" or cushion that normally is between the joint socket and the jaw joint.

CROWN (cap). *Anatomical crown* refers to the part of the tooth that is seen above the gums.

1. A dental restoration made of *acrylic, gold,* or *porcelain.* Cemented on damaged part of the natural tooth, called an anatomical crown.
2. Crowns that are made of metal may have any of the following compositions. The percentage is based on amount of gold present:

    high noble—Gold (Au), Palladium (Pd), and/or Platinum (Pt) > sixty percent (with at least forty percent Au);

    noble—Gold (Au), Palladium (Pd), and/or Platinum (Pt) > twenty-five percent;

    predominantly base—Gold (Au), Palladium (Pd), and/or Platinum (Pt) < twenty-five percent

CROWN LENGTHENING. If a tooth is cracked below the gum line, crown-lengthening exposes needed tooth structure surgically, in order for a crown to be made for it.

CURETTAGE. Removal of decayed or infected tissue. Used normally in dentistry during gum treatment for cleaning and removal of inflamed and infected gum tissue with advanced periodontal disease

CUSPID (see canine).

CYST. A sac filled with fluid or soft matter.

DDS. Doctor of Dental Surgery: degree given to dentists. Some dental schools designate the degree by DDS, others by DMD. Both represent the same level of professional education.

DMD. Doctor of Medical Dentistry (see above).

DECAY. Decomposition or destruction of tooth structure.

DELTA SLEEP. Stage(s) of sleep in which EEG delta waves are prevalent or predominant. Delta waves are constituted by EEG activity with a frequency less than 4 Hz. In human sleep stage scoring, conventionally the minimum criteria for scoring delta waves is 75 uV (peak-to-peak) amplitude, and 0.5 second duration (2 Hz).

DENTAL FLUOROSIS. A condition that results from drinking overly fluoridated water that often causes the teeth to become discolored and the enamel of the teeth to look spotted, pitted, or stained.

DENTAL IMPLANT. Device placed surgically in bone of the upper or lower jaw to support a dental restoration or prosthesis, to replace missing teeth.

DENTIN. Layer of tooth structure directly under enamel, or outer layer.

DENTURE. *Full Denture* is artificial replacement by a removable prosthetic when all teeth are missing. *Partial Denture* is artificial replacement by a removable prosthetic when some but not all teeth are missing. *Immediate Denture* refers to a denture that is placed in the mouth, immediately following extraction of teeth. *Overdenture* is a denture made to fit over implants or roots of teeth for support or better fit.

DESENSITIZING THERAPY. The process of reducing sensitivity by measured exposure to an allergen or stressor.

DIASTIMA. Space between teeth.

DIGITAL X-RAY. A very low radiation exposure technology by which X-rays of teeth can be viewed immediately by computer.

DISTAL. Facing the back of the dental arch, away from the midline.

DOXYCYCLINE. An antibiotic derived from tetracycline that is effective against many infections.

DRY MOUTH. Condition of the mouth with little or no moisture brought about by disease, radiation, anxiety, medication, and other causes.

DRY SOCKET. Inflammation due to infection or incomplete clotting in the socket after extraction (pulling) of a tooth.

EDENDULOUS. Missing all the teeth.

ENAMEL. The outer layer of the tooth on the crown portion.

ENDODONTIST. Dentist who specializes in the treatment of injuries to the pulp (chamber that houses the blood and nerve supply of the teeth).

EQUILIBRATION. Systematically adjusting tooth surfaces to even out the bite (occlusion).

EXOSTOSIS (see Torus).

EXPLORER. Instrument used to detect cavities.

FAGD. Fellow of the Academy of General Dentistry.

FEVER BLISTER (see cold sore).

FIBROMYALGIA SYNDROME (FMS). A chronic disorder that causes widespread pain and tenderness in the muscles and soft tissue as sleep problems, fatigue, and a variety of other symptoms.

FISTULA. A route or channel of drainage made near a tooth in the gums to drain infectious pus (gum boil). May not be accompanied by pain, but must be treated or could be life-threatening if the pus travels to the lungs, etc.

FLUORIDE. A trace mineral also known as fluorine. It's found in nature, but never alone, because it is a reactive element.

FLUORIDE TOOTHPASTE. Toothpaste containing fluoride, a trace mineral and is also known as fluorine. It's found in nature, but never alone, because it is a reactive element.

FLUOROSIS. A condition that results from ingesting too much fluoride, often causing the teeth to become discolored and the enamel of the teeth to look spotted, pitted, or stained.

FRENUM. The thin muscle tissue that attaches the tongue to the floor of the mouth, and the upper and lower lips to the gums. If the frenum is abnormally placed, *frenectomy* is performed to surgically re-shape or remove it.

GENERAL ANESTHESIA (see anesthetic).

GINGIVA. Gum tissue.

GINGIVAL HYPERPLASIA. An overgrowth of gingival tissues.

GINGIVECTOMY. Surgical removal of gum tissue.

GINGIVITUS. Inflammation of gum tissue.

GINGIVOPLASTY. Surgical reshaping and contouring of gum tissue to enhance function or appearance.

GLASS IONOMER. Dental material containing ground glass (polyalkenoate), used as a base liner under fillings or crowns, or as a restoration.

GOLD CROWN (see Crown).

GRAFT. Natural or synthetic tissue or bone used to replace defects in the bone or gums

Allogenic Graft—Tissue transplantation from source that is genetically different from patient's cells, but of the same species (may be freeze-dried or irradiated).

Autogenous Graft—Tissue taken from one part of the person and transplanted in another part of the same person.

Homologous Graft—Tissue taken from another host and transplanted.

GUAIFENESIN. A drug that reduces the thickness and stickiness of mucous. It has also been found to aid in the excretion of uric acid in the urine.

GUAIFENESIN PROGRAM (see Guaifenesin protocol).

GUAIFENESIN PROTOCOL. A treatment regimen developed R. Paul St. Amand, M.D. and involving the uses of guaifenesin and special diet.

GUM RECESSION. Abnormal shrinkage of gum tissue from trauma or surgery.

GUTTA-PERCHA. A whitish rubber derived from the coagulated milky latex of the gutta-percha tree.

HALITOSIS. Bad breath.

HANDPIECE. Dental drill or tool used to clean, shape, fill teeth, etc.

HERPES SIMPLEX VIRUS. A herpes virus that affects the skin and nervous system.

HMO (same as DMO). Health Maintenance Organization or Dental Maintenance Organization is a dental health plan by which a person is assigned to a particular dental office. Profit to the office is based on number of patients seen and minimizing treatment.

HOMEOPATHY. A method of treating disease with small amounts of remedies that, in large amounts in healthy people, produce symptoms similar to those being treated.

HOT TOOTH. Used to refer to an extremely painful tooth that is difficult to numb, due to inflammation of the nerve tissue.

HYDROGEN PEROXIDE. Disinfecting solution used by dentists to treat gum infection or inflammation for a limited amount of time. Not recommended for long-term use or it may cause gum problems.

HYPOPNEA. Shallow breathing in which the air flow in and out of the airway is less than half of normal—usually associated with oxygen desaturation.

IMPACTED TOOTH. A tooth that is either fully or partially under bone or tissue and usually needs to be removed or exposed surgically.

IMPLANT (see dental implant).

IMPRESSION. Mold taken of the teeth to fabricate crowns or any prosthesis.

INCISORS. Term used to describe four front top and bottom teeth that are seen closest to the midline of the lips.

INLAY. A dental restoration that is made outside of the tooth, either in the dental office or by a laboratory, and then cemented or bonded into the tooth. Can be made of composite, porcelain, or gold. Usually covers one to three surfaces of a tooth.

INTRAORAL CAMERA. A small camera the dentist uses to project the image of a tooth onto a television or computer screen.

IRRITABLE BOWEL SYNDROME (IBS). A disorder that causes nerves that control the muscles in the GI tract to become too active. The GI tract becomes sensitive to food, stool, gas, and stress. Causes abdominal pain, bloating, and constipation or diarrhea.

IV SEDATION (see anesthetic).

JACKET. An all porcelain crown, usually made for the front teeth.

LABIAL. Pertaining to the side of teeth or mouth that facing the lips, or any area around the lips.

LAMINATE. A cosmetic acrylic or porcelain veneer made by a laboratory and bonded to the surface of a tooth.

LASER. Has limited use in dentistry at this time, except for gum surgery and teeth whitening.

LASER SURGERY. A form of surgery that uses a laser light source to remove diseased tissues or treat bleeding blood vessels. The laser may also be used for cosmetic purposes, including removal of wrinkles, tattoos, or birthmarks.

LAUGHING GAS (Nitrous Oxide). Inhalation agent (gas) used for sedation. Effect varies among individuals. Does not have any bearing on pain sensation; only helps lower anxiety.

LESION. An area of tissue that is diseased.

LINGUAL. Any area pertaining to the tongue or area of teeth facing the tongue.

LOCAL ANESTHETIC (see anesthetic).

LYSINE. An essential amino acid found in proteins; occurs especially in gelatin and casein.

MALIGNANT. Disease in tissue that has the capacity to spread to surrounding tissues.

MALOCCUSION. Imbalanced contact between upper and lower teeth, causing a misaligned bite.

MANDIBLE. Lower jaw.

MARGIN. Area of dental restoration that must form a tight seal to the tooth. If a tight seal is not made, bacteria can enter even slight openings (open margin) and cause decay. Proper seal may also aggravate the gingival and cause inflammation.

MARYLAND BRIDGE (see bridge).

MASTICATION. Action of chewing food.

MAXILLA. Upper jaw.

MESIAL. Facing the midline of the dental arch.

MOLARS. Chewing teeth located in the back of the dental arch. Usually three present in each quadrant, the very last one called "wisdom tooth."

MONILIASIS (Thrush, Candidiasis). Fungal infection that may occur after use of long-term antibiotic therapy. Not uncommon in the mouth.

MOUTH GUARD (Night Guard, Splint). Appliance made to prevent wear due to grinding or clenching of the teeth, or to treat malocclusion and other symptoms due to temporomandibular joint disorder (TMJ).

NSAID. Non-steroidal anti-inflammatory drug often used in dentistry.

NEUROTRANSMITTER. Any of a group of substances that transmit nerve impulses across a synapse.

NIGHT GUARD (see Mouth Guard).

NITROUS OXIDE (see Laughing Gas).

NOVACAINE. One of the first types of local anesthetic. No longer in use; replaced by more effective agents.

OCCLUSION. The relationship of the upper and lower teeth on closure and during chewing.

ONLAY. Laboratory-produced dental restoration that covers three to four surfaces or cusps of a tooth; may be made of acrylic, porcelain, or gold.

ORAL CAVITY. The mouth and all the structures associated with it.

ORAL HYGIENE. The maintenance of health in the mouth by process of cleanliness.

ORAL AND MAXILLOFACIAL SURGEON. Dental specialist who specializes in surgery of the mouth, jaw and face, including removal of teeth, tumors, fractures, and cosmetic reconstruction of the jaws and sometimes the face.

ORAL PATHOLOGIST. Dental specialist who diagnoses oral diseases.

ORTHODONTIST. Dental specialist who corrects misalignment of teeth.

OSSEOUS. Referring to the bone.

OSTEOPLASTY. Surgical contouring and modification of the bone.

OSTEOPOROSIS. A condition of decreased bone mass. This leads to fragile bones which are at an increased risk for fractures. In fact, it will take much less stress to an osteoporotic bone to cause it to fracture. The term "porosis" means spongy, which describes the appearance of osteoporosis bones when they are broken in half and the inside is examined.

OSTEOTOMY. Surgical cutting of bone.

OVERBITE. The overlapping of the front teeth vertically.

OVERJET. The overlapping of the front teeth horizontally.

PALATE. Hard or soft tissues of the roof of the mouth.

PALLIATIVE. Refers to temporary relief of pain, but not cure.

PANORAMIC RADIOGRAPH. X-ray that shows a panoramic view of upper and lower jaw.

PARASTHESIA. Temporary or permanent loss of sensation.

PARTIAL DENTURE (see denture).

PEDODONTIST or PEDIATRIC DENTISTRY. Dental specialist focusing on treatment of children.

PERIAPICAL. Referring to the location at the end of the root of a tooth. (PA) X-ray refers to radiograph revealing the end of the root of a tooth.

PERIODONTAL DISEASE. Gum disease; has four stages: Gingivitis, Mild, Moderate, and Advanced

PERIODONTAL POCKET. Destruction of gum attachments to the tooth, resulting in areas or "pockets" that are difficult to clean and in which bacteria thrive. Must be treated and professionally cleaned regularly.

PERIODONTAL SURGERY. Surgical treatment for cosmetic purposes or treatment of disease of the supporting structures of the teeth.

PERIODONTIST. Dental specialist involved with the treatment of the supporting structures of the teeth.

PERIODONTITIS. A dental disorder that results from progression of, involving inflammation and infection of the ligaments and bones that support the teeth.

PERMANENT TEETH. Adult teeth; a full set consists of thirty-two teeth, under normal conditions.

PIT. A small defect or area in a tooth that is usually seen on the occlusal (chewing) surfaces of the back teeth.

PLAQUE. Soft, sticky film, forming on all tooth surfaces and gums, containing bacteria and food debris. If not removed thoroughly, will result in gum disease and tooth decay.

POLYSOMNOGRAM. Continuous and simultaneous recording of physiological variables during sleep, i.e., EEG, EOG, EMG (the three basic stage scoring parameters), EKG, respiratory air flow, respiratory excursion, lower limb movement, and other electrophysiological variables.

PONTIC. Name given to artificial tooth used in a fixed or removable bridge used to replace missing teeth.

PORCELAIN CROWN (see crown).

PORCELAIN VENEER. A laboratory-produced thin layer of porcelain, made to be bonded to the face of a natural tooth for cosmetic purposes.

POST. Metal or acrylic rod, (pre-fabricated or fabricated by laboratory), cemented or bonded in a tooth to replace missing tooth structure. Helps provide retention for crowns.

PPO. Preferred Provider (Dental) Organization through which the dentist agrees to provide dental care at reduced fees.

PRECISION ATTACHMENT. Artificial devices used to keep dental prosthesis in place. Can be used to stabilize fixed or removable prosthetics.

PREMEDICATION. Use of certain prescribed medications prior to dental treatment.

PROGNOSIS. The perceived outcome of treatment.

PROGRESSIVE MUSCLE RELAXATION (PMR). A relaxation technique that involves alternating contractions with relaxation of various muscle groups. The aim of this strategy is to build awareness of muscle tension and then learn to control and relax those tense muscle groups at will, one at a time.

PROPHYLAXIS. Term used in the dental profession to refer to professional routine cleanings.

PROSTHESIS. Any artificial appliance used to replace body parts.

PROSTHODONTIST. Dental specialist who is involved with treatment of prosthesis for the mouth, and "complete reconstruction" of the mouth to correct bite and replace missing teeth.

PROVISIONAL FILLING. Temporary sedative filling material to help with inflammation of nerve tissue. May be left in place for up to six weeks.

PULP. The chamber of the tooth that houses the blood vessels and nerve.

PULPITIS. Inflammation of the pulp tissue.

PYORRHEA. Old name for periodontal (gum) disease.

PYROPHOSPHATES. Salts, or esters, of pyrophosphoric acid.

QUADRANT. The mouth or dental arch is divided into four sections, two in the maxilla and two in the mandible. An imaginary line extends from the front midline and extends back to the last tooth.

RADICULAR. Pertaining to the root of a tooth.

RELINE. Improving the fit of a full or partial denture by remolding and resurfacing the area that fits over the bone and gums with new material. May be done in the office or by a laboratory.

RESTORATION. Replacement of any part of a tooth with variety of materials.

ROOT. The portion of the tooth that is located in the alveolar bone (socket) and is attached to the gums by connective tissue.

ROOT CANAL THERAPY. Treatment of damaged or diseased pulp tissue of a tooth.

ROOT PLANING. Treatment of gum disease by thoroughly removing plaque, calculus, toxins, and diseased portions of the root surface.

ROOT RESECTION. Removal of a portion of a diseased root and keeping the remainder root(s) and natural tooth.

RUBBER DAM. Soft latex or non-latex material used to isolate a tooth from contamination and to prevent debris from entering the throat and being swallowed.

SALICYLATES. The salts, or esters, of salicylic acids, or salicylate esters of an organic acid. Some of these have analgesic and anti-inflammatory activities

SALIVA. Fluid in the mouth that provides lubrication and aids swallowing. Contains water, bacteria, enzymes, mucus.

SALIVA EJECTOR. A tube placed in the mouth during dental treatment for suctioning of water and saliva.

SALIVARY GLANDS. Glands that secrete saliva into the mouth from ducts located in the cheeks, under the tongue and lower jaw.

SCALING AND ROOT PLANING (SRP). Removal of plaque and calculus from entire tooth, including the root surface, using special hand instruments or ultrasonic devices.

SEALANT. Acrylic resin painted and bonded on clean chewing surfaces of teeth to prevent decay.

SEROTONIN. A neurotransmitter that mediates several important physiological functions including neurotransmission, gastrointestinal motility, hemostasis, and cardiovascular integrity.

SIALODICHOPLASTY. Surgical procedure to treat salivary glands.

SINUSITIS. Inflammation of the sinus.

SJORGREN'S SYNDROME. An autoimmune condition characterized by dryness of mucous membranes including the mouth.

SKELETAL FLUOROSIS. A condition that results from drinking overly fluoridated water that can cause damage to bones

SLEEP APNEA. Temporary interruption of sleep from blockage in airway.

SNORING. Noise produced during sleep owing to vibration of the soft palate and the pillars of the oropharyngeal inlet. Many snorers have incomplete obstruction of the upper airway, and may develop obstructive sleep apnea.

SODIUM FLUORIDE. Commonly used as a cavity-fighting agent in commercial toothpastes, a close chemical relative of sodium chloride, or ordinary table salt.

SODIUM LAURYL SARCOSINATE. A plant-derived member of the carboxylate group.

SODIUM LAURYL SULPHATE. A caustic detergent useful for removing grease; although commonly included in personal care items (shampoos and toothpastes, etc.) it can irritate skin and should not be swallowed.

SODIUM MONOFLUOROPHOSPHATE (MFP). A very strong form of fluoride that could cause damage to teeth and bones.

SOFT PALATE. Roof of the mouth.

SOMNOPLASTY. Commercial name for radiofrequency treatment of certain sleep disorders

SPACE MAINTAINER. Device made mostly for children, to maintain space designated for teeth, if teeth are lost prematurely.

SPLINT. Means used to stabilize, protect, or support structures in the mouth.

STANNOUS FLUORIDE. A compounded form of fluorine used to fluoridate toothpaste and mouth rinse.

STOMATITIS. Inflammation of the tissues of the mouth.

STUDY MODEL. Models of patient's teeth and tissues that are used by the dentist for diagnostic purposes and treatment planning.

SUPERNUMERARY TEETH. Extra teeth.

SUPPURATION. Pus; bacterial contaminated fluid in tissue.

TARTAR. Term commonly used for calculus, which is mineralized plaque. Cannot be removed by brushing, but must be removed professionally using special instruments.

TEMPOROMANDIBULAR JOINT. The area below the ear that involves the mechanism that helps with function of the lower jaw and includes the head of mandible (lower jaw) called the "condyle" and the socket, which is located at the base of the skull (temporal bond).

TEMPOROMANDIBULAR JOINT DISORDER (TMJ). Disorder and abnormal function of the jaw joints, along with other difficulties involving function of the jaw, often accompanied by pain.

TINNITUS. Sensation of a ringing, roaring, or buzzing sound in the ears or head; often associated with various forms of a hearing impairment.

TOOTH WHITENING (see bleaching).

TORUS (exostosis). Bony elevation seen on either side of the floor of the mouth or palate. This is common and no treatment is necessary unless it becomes irritated or interferes with placement of prostheses. Tori is the plural form of torus.

TRENCH MOUTH (see ANUG). Painful gum condition characterized by infection, foul breath, mouth sores, and loss of gum contour.

TRISMUS. Difficulty in opening or restricted opening of the jaw accompanied with muscle spasm and inflammation of the muscles of the jaw.

TWILIGHT SLEEP (see anesthetic—intravenous).

UCR. Usual, customary, and reasonable fees charged by the dentist.

ULTRA-SOUND. A diagnostic procedure that projects high-frequency sound waves into the body and changes the echoes into pictures (sonograms) shown on a monitor. Different types of tissue reflect sound waves differently. This makes it possible to find abnormal growths.

UNILATERAL. Pertaining only to one side.

UVULA. A hanging piece of tissue at the end of the soft palate and the entrance to the throat.

VENEER. Plastic or porcelain facing placed on teeth to change shape, color, contour, or position of a tooth cosmetically.

VERTICAL DIMENSION. Position and dimension between upper and lower teeth that can be measured. May change with wear, age, or need to be changed for function or esthetic reasons.

WHITENING (see bleaching).

WISDOM TEETH (Third Molars). The last molars in each quadrant of the mouth. Usually erupt between the ages of eighteen and twenty-five.

XEROSTOMIA. Decreased flow of saliva that produces dry mouth.

XYLITOL. A sweetener found in plants and used as a substitute for sugar; it is called a nutritive sweetener because it provides calories, just like sugar.

For Further Information

Fibromyalgia Treatment Center: an excellent resource for fibromyalgia, support groups, referrals, etc.
(310) 577-7510
www.guaidoc.com

American Dental Association (ADA): source for finding phone numbers of local dental societies and for dentist referrals.
(800) 621-8099

Local Dental Societies: phone numbers may be found in the yellow pages or by calling the American Dental Association (see above). Call local dental societies for dentist referrals or dentist complaints.

Local water fluoride content: the Web site of the Center for Disease Control and Prevention allows consumers in participating states to examine basic information about their water system, including the number of people served by the system and the

target fluoridation level. Current participating states are: Arizona, Colorado, Delaware, Florida, Georgia, Illinois, Indiana, Iowa, Maine, Massachusetts, Michigan, Minnesota, Nebraska, New Hampshire, Nevada, North Dakota, Oklahoma, Pennsylvania, and Wisconsin.
www.cdc.gov/oralhealth/data_systems/index.htm

Center for Disease Control and Prevention:
www.cdc.gov

American Pain Foundation: provides resources and help for management of chronic pain. (888) 615-PAIN (7246)
www.painfoundation.org

American Chronic Pain Association:
(800)-533-3231
www.theacpa.org

American Pain Society:
(847) 375-4715
www.ampainsoc.org

Local dental schools and the Salvation Army are excellent resources for low-cost dental treatment. Some hospitals offer free or low-cost dental clinics whose services are offered to children and adults through dental schools or local governments or churches.

References

Alternative Dentistry

1. Denholz, Melvin and Elaine. 1977. *How to Save Your Teeth and Your Money.* New York: Van Nostrand Reinhold, 12.
2. McGuire, Thomas. 1972. *The Tooth Trip.* New York: Random House, 2.
3. Voll, R. 1975. Twenty years of electroacupuncture diagnosis. *American Journal of Acupuncture,* March, 15–38. See also Voll, R. 1981. Electoacupuncture (EAV) Diagnostics and Treatment Results in Odontogenous Focal Events. *American Journal of Acupuncture,* 9,4, (Dec.) 293–302.
4. Fischer, Richard D. "Dentistry and Homeopathy: An Overview," *Journal of the American Institute of Homeopathy,* (Dec.), 78,4, 140–147.
5. Ernst E. Pittler M H. 1998. The effectiveness of acupuncture in treating acute dental pain: a systemic review. *Br Dent J* 184: 443–472.
6. Blom M, Dawidson I, Angmar-Månsson B. 1992. The effect of acupuncture on salivary flow rates in patients with xerostomia. *Oral Surg, Oral Med, Oral Pathol* 73: 293–298.

7. Bowsher D. 1990. Physiology and pathophysiology of pain. *Acupunct Med* VII: 17–20.
8. Macdonald A. 1990. Acupuncture analgesia and therapy— Part 2. *Acupunct Med* VIII: 44–49.

Burning Mouth

1. Brown R, Krakow AM, Douglas T, Chokki SK. 1997. "Scalded mouth syndrome" caused by angiotensin converting enzyme inhibitors. *Oral Surg Oral Med Oral Pathol Oral Radiol Endod* 83:665–7.
2. Epstein JB, Marcoe JH. 1994. Topical application of capsaicin for treatment of oral neuropathic pain and trigeminal neuralgia. *Oral Surg Oral Med Oral Pathol* 77:135–40.
3. Grushka M, Bartoshuk LM. 2000. Burning mouth syndrome and oral dysesthesias. *Can J Diagnos* June: 99–109.

Canker Sores

1. ___ *Cecil's Textbook of Medicine*, 21st Ed. (2000). Diseases of the Mouth and Salivary Glands. Reading, MA: Addison-Wesley, p. 2242.
2. Kunz, J. R. M. and Finkel, A. J. (Eds.) 1987. *Mouth and tongue.*
3. Balch, Phyllis and James F. *Prescription for nutritional healing,* 3rd Edition.

Cosmetics

1. Matis BA. 2003. Tray whitening: what the evidence shows. *Compendium of Continuing Education in Dentistry* Apr 24(4A):354–62.
2. Matis BA. Hamdan YS. Cochran MA. Eckert GJ. 2002. A clinical evaluation of a bleaching agent used with and without reservoirs. *Operative Dentistry* (Jan.–Feb.) 27(1):5–11.
3. Haywood, V. 2003. Frequently Asked Questions About Bleaching. *Compendium of Continuing Education in Dentistry,* Special issue: Tooth Whitening. (Apr.)24, 4A.

4. Munoz-Viveros, C. 2003. Tooth Whitening—Expert Roundup. *Compendium of Continuing Education in Dentistry,* Special issue: Tooth Whitening. (Apr.), 24, 4A.

Diet and Nutrition

1. *2001. PDR for Nutritional Supplements,* First Edition.
2. Watts TL. 1995. Coenzyme Q_{10} and periodontal treatment: Is there any beneficial effect? *Br Dent J* 178: 209–213.
3. Jensen ME, Harlander SK, Schachtele CF, et al. 1984. Evaluation of the acidogenic and antacid properties of cheeses by telemetric recording of dental plaque. In Eds JJ Hefferen, HM Koehler, and JC Osborn: *Food, Nutrition and Dental Health.* Vol. V. Park Forest South, IL: Pathotox.
4. Sakashita et al. 1997. Diet and discrepancy between tooth and jaw size in the Yin-Shang period of China. *American Journal of Physical Anthropology* 103(4):497–505.

Fluoride

1. Danielson C, et al. 1992. Hip fractures and fluoridation in Utah's elderly population. *Journal of the American Medical Association* 268(6): 746–748.
2. Rich C. 1966. Osteoporosis and fluoride therapy. *JAMA.* 196: 149.
3. Silverstone, L.M. Caries and remineralization. *Dent. Hygiene* 57 (5): 30–36
4. Stannard J, Rovero J, Tsamtsouris A, Gavris V. 1990. Fluoride content of some bottled waters and recommendations for fluoride supplementation. *J Pedod* 14:103—
5. Whitford GM. 1987. Fluorides in dental products: safety considerations. *Journal of Dental Research* 66 (5) 1056–1060.
6. Ripa LW. 1991. A critique of topical fluoride methods (dentifrices, mouth rinses, operator-, and self-applied gels) in an era of decreased caries and increased fluorosis prevalence. *J Public Health Dent* 51:23–41.
7. American Dental Association. *Accepted Dental Therapeutics.*

Gum Disease

1. Ridker P. et al. 2002. Comparison of C-reactive protein and low-density lipoprotein cholesterol levels in the prediction of first cardiovascular events. *N Eng J Med*, Vol 347 No. 20:1557.
2. Noack, Genco, Trevisan, et al. 2002. *Journal of Periodontology*, Sept, Vol.72 No. 9; 1221–1227.
3. I Brook, AE Gober. 1998. Persistence of group A beta-hemolytic streptococci in toothbrushes and removable orthodontic appliances following treatment of pharyngotonsillitis. *Archives of Otolaryngology—Head & Neck Surgery.* (Sept)., 124: 9 :993–995.
4. HC Hung, W Willett, A Merchant, BA Rosner, A Ascherio, KJ Joshipura. Joshipura KJ, 2003. Oral health and peripheral arterial disease. *Circulation*, 2003, 107, 8. 1152–1157. Boston, MA: Harvard Univ, Sch Dent Med, Dept Oral Hlth Policy & Epidemiol.
5. Web site for American Association of Periodontist.

How to Find a Dentist

1. CDC. *Guideline for disinfection and sterilization in health-care facilities: recommendations of CDC and the Healthcare Infection Control Practices Advisory Committee* (HICPAC). MMWR.
2. Ahtone J, Goodman RA. 1983. Hepatitis B and dental personnel: transmission to patients and prevention issues. *J Am Dent Assoc* 106:219–22.
3. Food and Drug Administration. 2000. *Guidance for industry and FDA reviewers: content and format of premarket notification [510(k)] submissions for liquid chemical sterilants/high level disinfectants.* Rockville, MD: US Department of Health and Human Services, Food and Drug Administration.
4. 1992. *JADA* March 123:46–54.

Cold Sores

1. Crumpacker CS, Guelic RM. 1999. Herpes simplex. In IM Freedberg et al., eds., *Fitzpatrick's Dermatology in General*

Medicine, 5th ed., vol. 2, 2414–2426. New York: McGraw-Hill, Inc.

2. Godfrey HR. 2001. A randomized clinical trial on the treatment of oral herpes with topical zinc oxide/glycine. *Alternative Therapy Health Medicine,* 7(3): 49–56.

Root Canals

1. Meining, George. 1993. *Root Canal Cover Up,* Bion Publishing.
2. Easlick K. 1984. An evaluation of the effect of dental foci of infection on health. *JADA* 42:615–686, 694–697.
3. Sigurdsson A, Stancill R, Madison S. 1992. Intracanal placement of Ca(OH)$_2$: A comparison of techniques. *J Endod* 18:367–370.
4. Barker, B.C.W., Parsons, K.C. and Williams, G.L. 1974. Anatomy of root canals. Permanent maxillary molar. *Aust. Dent. J.* 19: 46–50.
5. Ingle, J., Edward, E. and Beveridge. 1976. *Modern Endodontic Therapy.* 2nd Ed., 44.
6. Grossman L. 1982. Pulpless teeth and focal infection. *J Endodon* 8:S18–S24.
7. Educational material from the American Association of Endodontics.

Temporomandibular Joint Disorder (TMJ)

1. Morgan, DH; Hall, WP; and Vamvas, SJ. 1977. *Diseases of the Temporomandibular Apparatus. A Multidisciplinary Approach.* St. Louis: CV Mosby Co. 318–24.
2. Raustia, A. M. and R. T. Pohjola. 1986. Acupuncture compared with stomatognathic treatment for TMJ dysfunction. Part III: Effect of treatment on mobility. *Journal of Prosthetic Dentistry* 56(5): 616–23.
3. Risdon, F. 1933. Ankylosis of the temporomandibular joint. *JADA* 21:1933–7.
4. Rast, WC; Waldrep, AC; and Irley. WC. 1969. Bilateral temporomandibular joint arthroplasty. *J Oral Surg* 27:871–4.

Index

A page number in bold indicates a glossary entry.